How to Get Through Revalidation

Making the process easy

Peter Davies

BSc, MB ChB, Diploma of Primary Care Research, FRCGP
Former Appraisal Lead, NHS Calderdale
GP Principal, Keighley Road Surgery, Illingworth, Halifax
Elected Member, Calderdale Clinical Commissioning Group
Provost, Yorkshire Faculty, RCGP
Yorkshire Faculty Representative on Council, RCGP

D0219707

Radcliffe Publishing
London • New York

Radcliffe Publishing Ltd
33–41 Dallington Street
London
EC1V 0BB
United Kingdom

www.radcliffehealth.com

British Library Cataloguing in Publication Data

A catalogue record for this book is available from the British Library.

ISBN-13: 978 190891 159 9

The paper used for the text pages of this book is FSC® certified. FSC (The Forest Stewardship Council®) is an international network to promote responsible management of the world's forests.

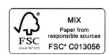

Typeset by Phoenix Photosetting, Chatham, Kent
Printed and bound by TJI Digital, Padstow, Cornwall

Contents

About the author

Peter Davies graduated from Leeds in 1989 and passed his Membership examination for the Royal College of General Practitioners (RCGP) and summative assessment in 1995. He became a GP principal at the Alison Lea Medical Centre in East Kilbride in 1996. In 2001, he moved back to his home town of Halifax. He worked as a salaried GP in the deprived area of Mixenden, Halifax, from 2001 to 2005, before moving as a partner to Keighley Road Surgery, Illingworth, Halifax, in 2005. He received his Fellowship of the RCGP in 2009.

Peter has many roles beyond his partnership – sometimes to the despair of his partners. He is provost of the Yorkshire Faculty of the RCGP, having previously been chair for many years. He represents the Yorkshire Faculty on the RCGP Council. He was GP Appraisal Lead for NHS Calderdale up to July 2012. He resigned this role so that he could concentrate on developing his work as Board Member of the Calderdale Clinical Commissioning Group.

He is a prolific and reflective medical author and has published many articles in the *BMJ*, *British Journal of General Practice* and elsewhere. He has written three previous books, entitled *Putting Patients Last* (Civitas, 2009), *The New GP's Handbook* (Radcliffe, 2012) and *Between Health and Illness – explorations in and around medicine* (Amazon Create Space and Kindle).

In this book, he is writing personally and not on behalf of any organisation.

He can be contacted via npgdavies@blueyonder.co.uk or via his Radcliffe Author page.

List of abbreviations

AOMRC	Academy of Medical Royal Colleges
BMA	British Medical Association
CCG	Clinical Commissioning Groups
CG	Clinical governance
CIR	Critical incident reporting
CPD	Continuing professional development
FTP	Fitness to practise
GMC	General Medical Council
GMP	Good Medical Practice
GMPGPs	Good Medical Practice for GPs
GPC	General Practitioners Committee
IDF	Independent Doctors Association
LMC	Local Medical Committee
MD	Medical director
MSF	Multiple source (colleague) feedback
MTPS	Medical Practitioners Tribunal Service
NASGP	National Association of Sessional General Practitioners
NCB	NHS National Commissioning Board
NHS	National Health Service
PCT	Primary care trust
PDP	Personal development plan
PSF	Patient source feedback
RCGP	Royal College of General Practitioners
RO	Responsible officer
SEA	Significant event audit
SUI	Serious untoward incident

Section 1

The overall architecture: who does what and when

Chapter 1

What this book is about

This book has been written to help ordinary regular doctors get through revalidation with grace and ease. When you have finished reading this book, you will understand the process properly, be much more relaxed about it and know exactly what you need to do to get through it.

The book is based on talks that my colleagues and I have given on this theme to several local audiences. Doctors are currently a bit scared about revalidation and as far as possible, I try to make the process simpler to understand and easier to achieve.

Revalidation has been discussed for many years – I think it was being mooted as far back as 1995 when I qualified as a GP. In fact, if you look further back, it was anticipated to some extent in *The Future General Practitioner* in 1972[1] and its early development is well described by Sir Donald Irving in *The Doctor's Tale*.[2] It has alternatively seemed either frightening or trivial, and it has raised spectres of doom such as '15% of doctors will fail revalidation'. Some of the medical magazines have tried hard to surpass the *Daily Mash*'s classic headline 'Everyone dead by teatime'. It has been difficult to get accurate information about the process mainly because the information has not been clear. Fortunately, cooler heads have prevailed. For example, a senior Local Medical Committee (LMC) officer commented about such stories, 'They can't be right. It'll be like medical finals – they can't fail too many of us at once as they've got a service to keep running'. In fact, it looks as if the 'failure rate' will be extremely low as most doctors are doing a decent job, and revalidation is about checking and confirming this.

Anyway, after a rather slow and tortuous journey,[3] revalidation is now ready to go and the process is at last clearly described. Jeremy

Hunt, the current Secretary of State for Health, has finally signed the relevant ministerial orders to authorise the General Medical Council (GMC) to run the process and so the process is now live.

You now have a specific legal duty to co-operate with this new process. This duty is about you as an *individual doctor*, not as part of your team. Therefore, in what follows, the message is personal and if any actions need to be taken, you yourself need to do them and make sure they are completed. Revalidation is your personal responsibility, not anyone else's. At the beginning and end of the day, it is *your* licence to practise medicine, and so *your* ability to earn money from *your* profession, that is at stake.

The purpose of revalidation is to show that you as a doctor are 'fit to practise and up to date'. The reason for the focus on doctors is simple. We are such a key part of the quality of the service experienced by patients that assuring the quality of doctors goes a long way towards ensuring the quality of the overall NHS service. So revalidation can be seen as part of the NHS's and the profession's efforts to raise levels of quality, performance and service.

Revalidation is about improving the service to patients. This book shows you how to demonstrate this and what information you will need to have available to satisfy your appraisers and responsible officers that you are fit to practise and up to date. Let me reassure you that it is much easier than you think – the process is not asking for that much information and you will (or should) have most of it to hand as part of your day-by-day practice of medicine. If you do not have it now, you should be able to gather it reasonably quickly.

So settle back, enjoy the book, understand the parts of revalidation and then look at your appraisal evidence and see what you need to add to it to be revalidation ready.

References

1   Royal College of General Practitioners. *The Future General Practitioner*. London: Royal College of General Practitioners; 1972.
2   Irvine D. *The Doctor's Tale: professionalism and public trust*. London: Radcliffe Publishing; 2003.
3   Pringle M. *Revalidation of Doctors –The Credibility Challenge*. John Fry Fellowship Lecture. London: Nuffield Trust; 2005.

Chapter 2
Your licence to practise medicine

In the old days, you got your licence to practise from the General Medical Council at full registration and then, provided you kept your nose clean, you and your employers could assume it was intact for your whole career.

These days you get your licence to practise and, after sufficient recognised postgraduate training, an entry on the appropriate specialist register. You also come under a local clinical governance (CG) process and a local continuing professional development (CPD) and appraisal system. The local medical director (MD) is at the apex of this system, monitoring its outputs. This relationship to a medical director is a new feature of the UK medical landscape in both hospital and primary settings that has emerged in the last 10 years or so.

As a doctor, your licence to practise is your *most valuable asset*, both for your professional pride and for your ability to earn a living from medicine. It can only be removed by the General Medical Council for a specific, legally valid reason. Failure to take part in the revalidation process is now a potential route to the GMC removing your licence. It is this risk that gives revalidation its teeth but removal of your licence is extremely unlikely if you know how to navigate the process successfully.

Like any asset, your licence to practise medicine comes with a *maintenance cost*. You need to accept this maintenance cost; your practising privileges are granted on condition that you will pay heed to the need to maintain your licence. Alternatively, I could say that it is now a clear part of your role and duty as a doctor to show that you maintain yourself in a fit state of intellectual and professional relationship development so that you are currently able to do your job well.[1,2] Your hard-earned medical degrees and college memberships from many years ago are not current evidence for this.

You will already be very busy seeing patients, and with the many other activities and bits of work that accrue around this clinical work. You need to know that you are doing this well and in accordance with current standards and guidance. This means that at certain times you will need to break off from your busy-ness and see how well you are actually doing your business. This is in sharp contrast to the old days when doctors were always busy – far too busy to interrupt this often unreflective business for any reason. Time out of surgery or hospital clinics to undertake such reflective work should now be a routine part of normal clinical practice, and it should be counted as work or study leave, not as time off. Surgeries and hospital departments should be planning time for learning and reflection into the working pattern of every doctor, and they should be keen to hear the results from each individual doctor's learning and audits. In Peter Senge's phrase, clinical teams need to be functioning as 'learning organisations'.[3] Currently some achieve this and some do not.

It is your responsibility as an individual doctor to pay willingly the costs of keeping your licence intact. If you are not willing to pay this cost then you deservedly run the risk that your licence will not be renewed. If professional status means anything, it is a permanent and perennial concern about how well you do your job.

Once you show signs of not caring about the quality of your work or not owning the results of your actions, you cease to really be a professional. You become a hollow mockery of a professional. You could, in Raymond Tallis's memorable phrase,[4] degenerate into a 'sessional functionary robotically following guidelines'.

To be professional is to be perennially self-critical, to always reflect on your actions and their outcomes, to always be learning and to have a boundless curiosity that drives you to keep learning more. Once you are reduced to 'I only work here', 'That's the way it is round here' or 'I'm always busy', you have given up a part of your professional status and your stature is reducing.

In many ways, a defining feature of professionalism is that your internal standards are so high that it becomes unnecessary and even counterproductive to supervise your work. In the old days of medicine, this view was probably taken too far. Nowadays, your basic abilities will be accepted but you may well be negotiating about where and to what purpose they need to be deployed. It is called job planning or, in general practice, a discussion about the varying merits of internal and external income streams.

Taking part in CPD and appraisal pays the cost of maintaining your licence to practise. The hope is that in the future, the work you do personally as CPD will also help with input into area-wide service improvements as part of commissioning and service improvement leadership. If things work out well, then our individual and collective efforts should become part of one whole.

References

1 General Medical Council. *Good Medical Practice*. London: GMC; 2006. Available at: www.gmc-uk.org/static/documents/content/GMP_0910. pdf (accessed 30 November 2012).
2 Royal College of General Practitioners. *Good Medical Practice for General Practitioners*. London: Royal College of General Practitioners; 2008. Available at: www.rcgp.org.uk/policy/rcgp-policy-areas/~/media/Files/ Policy/A-Z%20policy/Good_Medical_Practice_for_GPs_July_2008. ashx (accessed 30 November 2012).
3 Senge P. *The Fifth Discipline: the art and practice of the learning organization*. London: Century Business; 1990.
4 Tallis R. *Hippocratic Oaths: medicine and its discontents*. London: Atlantic Press; 2005.

Chapter 3

The overall architecture of revalidation

Revalidation is meant to be a routine output of local clinical governance processes and routine clinical activities. The process is overviewed here and then the individual chapters provide more specific detail about each part of the whole.

As a doctor, whether in hospital or in primary care, you are part of a local clinical governance process. Clinical governance processes have two main parts: educational and performance management.

The *educational processes* are formative and supportive. They are now moving towards being explicit and a core part of the NHS system (they were not always so in the past). The days of doctors feeling that they are 'good despite the system' should be going, and NHS organisations and private providers should include provision for staff development and training as an intrinsic part of their work. These days, doctors should be good because of the system they work within and the support it gives them to become better. The basic components of the educational channel are CPD and the appraisal system. Your appraisals confirm that you have a CPD strategy in place and are using it. These processes are fundamentally benign and concerns could only arise here if you were not making use of them. But why would you be so daft as not to take advantage of opportunities for CPD?

The *performance management processes* are those around performance concerns such as complaints, outlying measurements and maybe convictions. These are potentially more dangerous. Such concerns will be dealt with by the medical director as soon as they arise. They will not emerge as sudden and unexpected evidence at the time of the revalidation decision. You will already know about any such concerns. Record how you have dealt with such concerns as part of your appraisal process, partly for the record and partly to review what are potentially quite traumatic events in the supportive and educational process of appraisal. For revalidation purposes, the main requirement is that you have responded sensibly to such concerns by a reflective process leading to learning or an improvement in practice.

The responsible officer (RO) integrates the outputs from the educational and performance management systems, and can then make a well-evidenced recommendation to the GMC about your revalidation.

The RO can only really make three decisions and you as an individual doctor should know what your RO will decide. The RO regulations and the GMC's guidance about RO decision making are very specific, and basically divide the decisions they can make into three groups.

- If there are no performance concerns and your appraisals confirm satisfactory educational progress then the RO has no option but to revalidate you – hopefully more than 95% of us will be in this group.

- If there are issues around either unresolved performance concerns or incomplete revalidation evidence then revalidation will be deferred pending the resolution of concerns and completion of evidence gathering. This option leaves your licence to practise fully intact. Deferral is likely to be used in scenarios such as a complaint awaiting resolution or when a doctor has been on sickness or maternity leave for a long period and needs some time to catch up. Deferrals are for a specific period and for a specific reason. Minor complaints will not hold up an RO's revalidation decision. If a complaint raises a major issue (and the criterion for this would be an issue that is likely to constitute serious professional misconduct, in other words something that would be going through to GMC processes anyway), then the revalidation decision would pass to the GMC along with investigation of the complaint.

- If there is non-engagement with the revalidation processes then the RO will signal this to the GMC either as non-engagement itself or as a potential performance concern. However, as an individual doctor, you would have to be almost deliberately daft or foolhardy to end up in this group. And it is likely that such concerns would have drawn you to the RO's attention long before your revalidation decision is due. The processes are clear and it is a duty on you to co-operate with them. If you are not doing so, what standard is your practice at? Do you actually want to continue as a doctor and accept the obligations that high-standard professional work makes on you?

If your career is struggling or failing, this is likely to be picked up by the RO long before the revalidation decision. Appropriate help and support are likely to be mobilised for you before the date of revalidation. You will only run into trouble if you do not take the help offered. If the issue is a health concern then the ROs and the medical directors will try to get you help and support. The RO would much prefer to head off any trouble, for you and for them, if they can.

Responsible officers do not want to refer doctors to the GMC for non-engagement with the revalidation process but if they have to, they will. If you are sensible, you will make sure the thought of this action does not even cross your RO's mind in your case.

The GMC has set up specific procedures to deal with non-engagement. It is likely that your portfolio of supporting information would be reviewed at the GMC and you would be asked to complete any missing evidence within an agreed time frame. If you fail to do the remedial work then your licence can be withdrawn on the basis of your non-engagement with the process. To have reached this point, you would probably have ignored or failed to answer a mixture of encouragement and demands from appraisers and ROs for supporting information over time (possibly many years). To then ignore or fail to answer similar requests from the GMC would be reckless. In other words, to let your lack of appraisal and revalidation supporting information lead to such scrutiny would take deliberate inactivity on your part. It would not just happen.

Sadly, some doctors will let this happen to them and will fall at the revalidation hurdle. It seems a needless and pointless way to let anyone's medical career be ended.

The point of revalidation is not to suddenly uncover a lot of poorly performing doctors for the first time. If anything, the point of the process is that it forces local NHS organisations in hospital trusts and primary care, and outside employers in the private sector, to maintain good local clinical governance processes in action, that monitor the work of their doctors, deal with concerns earlier and support their doctors to do better. The days of doctors being good *despite* the system they work in should be going, and instead we should be able to say that we are good *because of* the systems we work within.

A recommendation for your revalidation is a positive statement about your ongoing high-quality performance as a doctor and should be appreciated as such.

The RO integrates the outputs from the educational and performance management channels and then makes their recommendation to the GMC. The GMC makes the final decision and lets you know the result. You carry on practising medicine well and wonder what you were worried about. Revalidation for most of us is about as interesting a process as renewing a library book, if rather more important.

Further reading

- GMC guidance on revalidation: www.gmc-uk.org/doctors/revalidation. asp (accessed 30 November 2012).

Chapter 4

The General Medical Council's role in revalidation

As a doctor, you have a licence to practise medicine from the GMC. This licence is granted by the GMC and can only be taken away from you by the GMC.

Your licence to practise medicine is a precious asset to you, both in terms of showing that you belong to the profession and in terms of your ability to earn a living from medical work. For most doctors, the thought of losing their licence to practise is one of their biggest fears.

In the past, you got your licence to practise medicine after graduation and provided you didn't end up in front of a Fitness to Practise Panel at the GMC, it stayed intact throughout your whole career.

The new rules mean that our licences to practise need to be revalidated once every five years. Revalidation is really a periodic examination of your continuing fitness to practise medicine. It is a quality control mechanism in medicine and is meant to protect the public from doctors whose performance might be putting their safety at risk.

More positively, it provides evidence to you, your patients and colleagues that your practice of medicine is along the right lines and sensibly directed. From the GMC's viewpoint, it is a way of ensuring that the advice and standards in *Good Medical Practice* are acknowledged and implemented. For us as doctors, the work needed for revalidation may help to keep our careers more focused and on track, and may actually strengthen us by providing clear evidence of ongoing high standards of performance. This may set up the virtuous cycle in which being revalidated may justifiably make us feel better about the quality of our work, which encourages us to do better in the future. This may both reduce our risk of complaints and achieve better results for patients. At the very least, if a complaint comes in, it will be seen as an isolated blip rather than yet more evidence of permanent, persistent and pervasive failings in our practice.

Think about this old scenario, which was seen at the GMC too many times in earlier years. A patient submitted a complaint about a 55-year-old GP to the GMC. The GMC investigated the allegation. The GP worked in a single-handed setting. Their medical degree came from abroad, and some time ago. There was not much local knowledge of this particular doctor or his work. It was difficult to know whether the index complaint was an isolated incident or an ongoing pattern of poor performance. There was no-one at the health authority who was responsible for gathering such information reliably and systematically, and so there was no-one who could give the GMC any reliable local intelligence about the doctor. The complaint was about the doctor's manner, and alleged rudeness and also some medical incompetence. On further investigation, the complaint turned out to be the tip of an iceberg and further evidence emerged of failings in that doctor's attitude and manner. The case ended up being substantial, and progressed to a Fitness to Practise Panel. The doctor had difficulty mounting a defence and so then ended up being erased from the Register on the grounds that he had shown serious professional misconduct. In more modern terms, he would have been shown to be in breach of the principles of *Good Medical Practice*, and posing an ongoing risk to the safety of patients.

Now what would happen in this scenario if the GP had been actively taking part in his appraisals and providing evidence of ongoing thought and reflection about his work? If he had looked at complaints as they arose, and thought about what he was doing well and not so well and adjusted his medical practice accordingly? If he had been revalidated only two years earlier? If there was a local system of performance monitoring managed by the local medical director? It would be much harder for the doctor now to be erased or even charged. There would be strong evidence of at least reasonable prior standards of performance. There would be evidence of ongoing critical engagement with and reflection on his work. The index complaint could more easily be seen as an isolated example, rather than as part of a pattern of poor performance. It would be much easier for the GP to mount a decent reply and defence to the complaint. Imagine meeting a complaint about your manner with 'I'm sorry to hear that. It's unusual for me. Here is the result of my patient feedback from last year and it shows me usually performing well at this'. You would be on very solid ground indeed. Revalidation in such a case would indeed have made you strong again.

The GMC is responsible for revalidation and makes the decisions about the revalidation of individual doctors. However, the GMC is relying on a network of locally based responsible officers to gather the information it needs to make its decision. In practice, this means that the decision about revalidation is largely made by the RO, with the GMC basically agreeing with it. Technically, the RO recommends that an individual doctor should be revalidated and the GMC decides. It seems unlikely that in practice the GMC will change or challenge many of an RO's recommendations.

The GMC will quality assure the work of the ROs and make sure they operate to consistent standards. However, it is unlikely that the GMC will change the recommendations from individual ROs unless there is suspicion of a significant mistake having been made, or additional information has emerged. And the ROs are too careful to let that happen.

For you as an individual, there is one action you need to take now. You need to register at GMC Online (www.gmc-uk.org/doctors/information_for_doctors/gmc_online.asp) and link yourself to your RO. This sets up the chain doctor–RO–GMC, so that your revalidation recommendation can go through easily.

The GMC issues the most authoritative guidance about the evidence required for revalidation, and it is worth reading this. It is summarised in the relevant places in this book.

Further reading

- GMC guidance on revalidation: www.gmc-uk.org/doctors/revalidation. asp (accessed 30 November 2012).

Chapter 5

The responsible officer's role in revalidation

The ROs are the key players in the revalidation process. They are senior doctors who are usually employed as medical directors, and who have significant experience of managing the performance of doctors. They are at the apex of the revalidation process and are basically making the decision, although formally they make a recommendation to the GMC which then says 'We agree with the RO'.

The RO is in post to make sure that local educational, appraisal and performance management procedures work well. Their role is very procedurally bound and is defined in the Responsible Officer Regulations issued by the Department of Health in January 2011.

Responsible officers must act on the basis of evidence, and free from personal prejudices. If there is a personal issue that could affect their decision, they will acknowledge the conflict of interest (whether actual or potential) and ask for help from another RO.

The RO has three basic decisions they can make about your revalidation.

- If they know that the educational processes are in place and there are no performance concerns then they must revalidate you. The ROs are hoping that at least 95% of doctors fall easily into this group.

- If they know of unresolved performance concerns, health issues such as long-term sickness absence or prolonged maternity leave then they can defer your revalidation pending provision of the additional evidence needed to make a properly informed revalidation decision. Such a deferral will be for a defined period and for a specific reason.

If you end up being deferred, make sure you use the extra time to get the necessary information together quickly. It is a bit like an extension to a deadline on a university project – you are welcome to it but not to a further one.

- If you have not engaged with the processes of clinical governance, whether performance management or educational, then you are putting your status on the performers list, and maybe your GMC registration, in jeopardy. You would be doing this yourself, and it would be no good blaming anyone other than yourself for this outcome. If an RO picks up evidence of non-engagement they will treat it as a performance concern, and this places your licence to practise at risk. They will deal with non-engagement as it arises, and before your revalidation decision is due.

What evidence does the responsible officer need?

We have now the basic architecture of the RO's role. But this then leads to the question of what evidence the RO will need to see to be able to make a fair and accurate decision about a doctor's revalidation.

First, the RO will review the evidence from performance management procedures. This evidence is already available within hospital trusts or primary care trusts (PCTs) and their successor bodies such as the NHS Commissioning Board and its local outposts.

Second, they will review a summary of the evidence provided at appraisal. The RO will not have time to read all your appraisals even in summary. They will be relying on their appraiser teams to provide the information to them in a highly condensed format, which basically needs to confirm that the appraisal has happened and that the specific supporting information needed (as specified by the GMC requirements) has been checked and found to be satisfactory by the appraiser. Assuming they are assured on this, they can then make a fair decision about revalidation.

Your RO is best viewed as an intelligent and respected senior colleague, and not encountered when their investigatory antennae have been alerted.

Role of your appraiser

So your appraiser has a key role here to know what the RO needs to see and to help make sure their doctors being appraised have provided this to them.

Remember that although your appraiser will help you with advice, encouragement, provocation and whatever stimulus you need, it is ultimately your responsibility as an individual doctor to provide the relevant evidence when it is needed. The supporting structures will try and nudge you to the right actions ... *but you need to perform the action.*

Ultimately, this book is all about letting you know what you need to do to get revalidated. There is a team of colleagues around you who can help you. If you take the advice in this book on board then you will find the process smooth and straightforward, and make your RO's decision very easy and favourable to you. If you try to take your own route then you risk losing your licence to practise and your ability to earn a living.

Further reading

- Department of Health. *The Medical Profession (Responsible Officers) Regulations 2010.* London: Department of Health; 2010. Available at: www.legislation.gov.uk/uksi/2010/2841/made (accessed 30 November 2012).
- General Medical Council. *Ready for Revalidation: making revalidation recommendations: the GMC responsible officer protocol.* London: General Medical Council; 2012. Available at: www.gmc-uk.org/static/documents/content/Responsible_Officer_Protocol.pdf (accessed 30 November 2012).

Chapter 6

The appraiser's role in revalidation

Over the last 10 years doctors and appraisers have got used to the appraisal interview as a formative reflective process. This has been a wide-ranging reflective interview and conversation. Sometimes it has been useful for the doctor being appraised and sometimes it has not. But fundamentally, it has been formative and developmental and when done well, it should have helped the doctor being appraised to adjust their practice of medicine and encourage them to make the changes necessary for them to practise medicine better and so help their patients more.

As appraisers, we have tried to make the appraisal discussions rooted in evidence, as opposed to unrooted and unanchored commentary. The terminology has now moved from 'evidence' to 'supporting information'.

We have been up against some doctors who are so overconscientious that they supply more than one lever arch file full of supporting information and ask 'Is this enough?'. We have been up against some minimalist doctors who wrote one cryptic sentence under each of the old appraisal headings and wondered if they could have been briefer. We have been up against some doctors who provided no evidence at all. We have been up against some anxious and fearful doctors, for whom any review of their practice is an event provoking great dread.

We have regularly tried to get our appraisees to bring enough evidence about their work to help the discussion, and to keep that evidence relevant and personal to them and not just the practice manager's bundle of 'evidence for appraisal'.

We have long tried to get our appraisees to go beyond just flinging information at us, and instead to focus on their reflection on the outcomes – namely what they have done, what they have learned, and what they will do better in the future as a result of that reflection.

All such questions about what, and how much, to bring to appraisal are now going to be redundant. The GMC's requirements for appraisal now make it very clear what supporting information needs to be brought to appraisal and reflected upon. The headings now are:

- quality improvement activity

- significant event audits

- continuing professional development

- patient source feedback (PSF)

- multiple source (colleague) feedback (MSF)

- response to concerns and compliments.

So this rather circumscribes what your appraiser wants to see. The appraisal interview may well involve much interesting conversation, about many topics. But in terms of what has to be included, the six headings above cover it.

Revalidation-ready appraisees will make sure that the supporting information under these headings is present and has been reflected upon, and that the appraiser can reassure the RO that the educational processes of evidence gathering and reflection have occurred. We will be moving to evidence-rooted appraisals. Provided the supporting information is present, the discussion will continue to be a formative, supportive and, usually, enjoyable developmental process. If, however, there is a lack of evidence, the summative side will come in, with MDs and ROs becoming worried about 'lack of engagement with the process'.

I need to say here that not every heading needs to be covered each year. However, over the five-year revalidation cycle, you need some relevant evidence under each heading reflecting the full scope of your professional practice. Your appraisals over time should be recording the gathering of a relevant portfolio of evidence.

For those of us who have many roles, it will pay us to have supporting information under each heading for each role, gathered over time. For example, a Clinical Commissioning Group (CCG) member might have a quality improvement project as part of their CCG work in one year and a clinical audit of an activity at the surgery the next. For the appraiser and RO, the key here is that there is evidence of concern about quality improvement. The whole portfolio can be gathered steadily over five years, to fully reflect the scope of work.

For you as a doctor being appraised, these headings make life simpler for you. Is your audit project relevant evidence? Yes of course it is. Is your essay on how you get on with your colleagues relevant? Not really, but we would love to see your MSF and see what you have learned from it. It gives us better evidence and allows you and us to see how much match or mismatch there is between your view of yourself and your colleagues' view of you.

The old days of reflective commentaries are going. Coming in is the need for specific bits of information. As your appraisal is approaching, think about gathering the specific evidence required for it. And gather evidence that as far as possible is *personal to you* and not merely the practice or departmental file.

We know you cannot be totally separated from your context of work. However, revalidation is about your individual practice of medicine and not about the group you belong to.

The role of the appraiser in revalidation is to make sure that appraisees are gathering and reflecting on relevant supporting information that over the five-year cycle builds into a portfolio that makes the RO's decision about their revalidation easy and favourable to them.

Paying attention to last year's appraisal

Part of appraisal is a review of progress against last year's objectives. So the appraiser does need to see last year's appraisal summary and personal development plan (PDP) and to formally note progress against last year's goals.

The appraisal summary

One of the key roles of the appraiser is to produce a summary of the appraisal discussion. In the old days this was known as 'Form 4'. It is now just called the appraisal summary. It is an important document for you and for your RO. The appraisers take pride in getting this document right.

Mostly it is factual and will say things such as 'I saw the evidence of an audit about cholesterol management. The audit showed evidence gathering, reflection, and some specific actions have been taken in the light of its findings'. There will then be a statement about which of the domains and attributes of *Good Medical Practice* this provides evidence for.

The summary is now written under the headings of *Good Medical Practice*. The four domains are:

1 knowledge, skills and performance

2 safety and quality

3 communication, partnership and teamwork

4 maintaining trust.

Each domain has three attributes.

- Knowledge, skills and performance

1 Maintain your professional development.

2 Apply knowledge and experience to practice.

3 Keep clear, accurate and legible records.

- Safety and quality

1 Systems to protect patients and improve care.

2 Respond to risks to patient safety.

3 Protect patients from risks posed by your health.

- Communication, partnership and teamwork

1 Communication skills.

2 Work constructively with colleagues; delegation.

3 Establish and maintain partnerships with patients.

- Maintaining trust

1 Show respect for patients.

2 Treat patients fairly and without discrimination.

3 Act with honesty and integrity.

One of the purposes of appraisal and revalidation is to make the principles of *Good Medical Practice* relevant in practice. This new way of producing the appraisal summary ties it very closely into *Good Medical Practice*.

There are five statements to be made at the end of the appraisal discussion by the appraiser to the RO.

1 An appraisal has taken place that reflects the whole of the doctor's scope of work and addresses the principles and values set out in *Good Medical Practice. Agree/Disagree*

2 Appropriate supporting information has been presented in accordance with the *Good Medical Practice* framework for appraisal and revalidation and this reflects the nature and scope of the doctor's work. *Agree/Disagree*

3 A review that demonstrates progress against last year's personal development plan has taken place. *Agree/Disagree*

4 An agreement has been reached with the doctor about a new personal development plan and any associated actions for the coming year. *Agree/Disagree*

5 No information has been presented or discussed in the appraisal that raises a concern about the doctor's fitness to practise. *Agree/Disagree*

The appraiser should record any comments that will assist the RO to understand the reasons for the statements that have been made.

As you can see from all this, the appraiser has a thorough matrix of concepts against which to work. Thus, you as the doctor being appraised and ultimately revalidated now know how to make their job easier.

Further reading

- General Medical Council. *Ready for Revalidation: making revalidation recommendations: the GMC responsible officer protocol.* London: General Medical Council; 2012. Available at: www.gmc-uk.org/static/documents/content/Responsible_Officer_Protocol.pdf (accessed 30 November 2012).

Chapter 7

The individual doctor's role in appraisal and revalidation

Statutory requirements

It is *your* licence to practise, isn't it? It is an asset to you, isn't it? Both in terms of confirming your professional standing, and in terms of your ability to earn your living. In other words, the most crucial person in revalidation is *you*, the individual doctor. You are fit to practise and up to date, aren't you?

However you look at it, revalidation is about you and up to you. You can either accept the process and work with it or you can try resisting it, but like Arthur Dent lying down in front of the bulldozer, your actions will be futile and the new hyperspace bypass will simply blast past you.[1] The process is now mandatory with legal force behind it. This creates a duty you need to fulfil if you want to keep your licence to practise medicine intact.

The basic requirement on you as an individual undergoing revalidation is to keep attending your appraisals and providing relevant supporting information for them. If there are concerns about your performance or complaints, deal with them courteously and review them at the appraisal interview.

The positive route through this

However, I would encourage you to look on all this in a positive light and to see the opportunity it provides to you. The revalidation and appraisal processes partly have a duty to guide your work, and partly a positive duty to support your continuing professional development.

As Matt Walsh, Colin Pollock and I put it in a *British Journal of General Practice* paper in 2011: 'The days of doctors being "good despite the system" should be going, and instead we should be able to say that doctors are good because of the system they work in'.[2]

Appraisal and revalidation processes represent the systematic attempts of the NHS and the GMC to help you with your ongoing professional development, either encouraging your existing efforts or reminding and encouraging you to do better. They are basically educational, and they are the first consciously created system to look at supporting doctors in an educational and to some extent pastoral manner.

Appraisal is not itself pastoral but if problems are found earlier because of reflection during appraisal, then help and support can be mobilised before the problems become more major and cause damage either to the doctor's reputation or abilities or to any patients. One of the benefits of appraisal may be that it is allowing problems to be dealt with at an early stage when education and other supports are sufficient, and before the problem becomes worse and then the doctor has to be dragged into the disciplinary processes or a partnership dispute. It is probably impossible to quantify this claim but at the very least, for doctors the appraisal process allows some time out for reflection and an opportunity to head problems off.

Appraisal is the first attempt by the NHS at any process of maintenance for the important asset that is medical professionals. In the old days (from 1948 to about 2002), it was largely assumed that professionals would maintain themselves and that the 'odd failure or two' was acceptable attrition. This led to a phenomenon of battle-hardened cynical older doctors who were often in post as much for their ability at bluffing and toughing out the NHS as their clinical abilities.[3] Doctors who remained or became good doctors in such a system were good largely because of some inner personal resilience rather than because they worked in a system that made them good. Indeed, they were often good despite the system they worked within, and as a result often somewhat contemptuous of that system. Their retirement interviews often carried a 'Goodbye to all that' flavour about them.[4-7]

In other words, the NHS now cannot simply say 'You are a consultant surgeon and that's what you will do until you retire'. The CPD processes are about our evolution as professionals through our careers, and are beginning to recognise the need for change and adaptation within our jobs. The CPD reflected in the appraisal process may pave the way for our jobs to alter and adapt through time as we change, and as medical knowledge increases and NHS structures change. Ask a 65-year-old surgeon what he would say to his 35-year-old self when he was newly appointed, or to a newly appointed colleague. Or as a consultant put it to me, 'I thought I knew what I was going to be doing when I was appointed. Now I find I'm doing that and a whole lot of things I never thought I would have to be doing'.

Approached positively, the CPD, appraisal and revalidation process is a support structure for your ongoing adaptation to change in your work. If you use it positively then it will help you do better personally and for patients and for your local part of the system.

Remember that the process is continuous. The appraisal interview is a periodic review, not the end or purpose of the process. Revalidation is basically a check that you are following some sort of CPD strategy (in other words, there is evidence of a plan or purpose to the learning activity) and that you are not getting too many complaints or concerns.

For most doctors, revalidation is not a major hurdle, and the specific pieces of evidence the GMC requires for revalidation should be easy enough to gather.[7] The requirements and their justification are described in the following chapters.

Key points about your involvement in your appraisal

- Own your appraisal – this is an opportunity for you.

- It's a continuous process and not just an interview once a year.

- Keep it personal – it's about you, not them.

- A small amount of personally relevant material with reflection, learning points and action points is what the appraisers want to see.

- Revalidation is a minor event but one that reflects and confirms that important underlying professional processes are in place.

- The system and those of us running it want you to perform well and to help you maintain that high standard.

- All the appraisal and CPD activity you do is ultimately about improving the service you can provide to patients.

Appraisal is a professional obligation. Not taking part risks your status on the list and thereby your licence to practise. More positively, appraisal is an opportunity to reflect on your work, and a system that will help you to do it better in the future, increasing your satisfaction and enjoyment, and it is to your patients' benefit.

Engaging with revalidation is a simple decision: if you keep your CPD and appraisals up to date and avoid performance management issues, the RO, whoever he or she is, has to recommend you for revalidation.

The appraisal evidence headings and the questions being asked of you are as follows.

- Continuing professional development – What am I doing to keep up to date and to improve?

- Quality improvement activity – What are my current standards of practice like?

- Significant event audit (SEA) – What do I do about unusual events?

- Multiple source feedback (MSF) – How do I come across to my colleagues?

- Patient feedback (PF) – How do I come across to my patients?

- Response to complaints and concerns – How have I handled concerns about my work?

The emphasis throughout is on demonstrating reflection and learning, and actions taken in response to identified problems. The appraiser's job is to help you get that process of reflection right, and to focus it into useful educational activities that meet your educational needs.

The appraisal process is about the individual doctor. The hope is that, in the future, the work you do as CPD will also help with input into area-wide service improvements as part of commissioning. If things work out well then our individual and our collective efforts should become part of one whole.

Structuring your evidence for appraisal

One of the purposes of appraisal and revalidation is to encourage doctors to understand the principles of *Good Medical Practice* more easily and thoroughly. It is worth reminding ourselves here about the domains and attributes of *Good Medical Practice*. One smart way of considering evidence for appraisal is to ask yourself which of these domains and attributes your appraisal evidence shows in action. To remind you, the four domains are:

1 knowledge, skills and performance

2 safety and quality

3 communication, partnership and teamwork

4 maintaining trust.

Each domain has three attributes.

- Knowledge, skills and performance

1 Maintain your professional development.

2 Apply knowledge and experience to practice.

3 Keep clear, accurate and legible records.

- Safety and quality

1 Systems to protect patients and improve care.

2 Respond to risks to patient safety.

3 Protect patients from risks posed by your health.

- Communication, partnership and teamwork

1 Communication skills.

2 Work constructively with colleagues; delegation.

3 Establish and maintain partnerships with patients.

- Maintaining trust

1 Show respect for patients.

2 Treat patients fairly and without discrimination.

3 Act with honesty and integrity.

Over the five-year revalidation cycle, ideally your portfolio will contain examples of each of these attributes being enacted. Of course, one piece of evidence can show multiple attributes.

Weaknesses of the appraisal system

There are some significant weaknesses to the appraisal system, and it is worth bearing these in mind.[8]

The first is a cognitive flaw we all have: we tend to gild the lily in areas we already know well and miss the gaps in our knowledge of other areas. In appraisal, the doctor being appraised presents positive evidence of what they have done and why, and the appraiser properly pays attention to this. What goes unsaid by the appraisee, and is often unnoticed by the appraiser, is where the areas of weakness and ignorance lie. Very few of us are aware of our areas of ignorance.[9] If we were, we would have done something about them! Appraisal does not have a system within it to pick up on these. We do not know that which we do not know – this is the famous Dunning–Kruger effect.[10] The advent of MSF and PSF does now bring the perspective of the other into the discussion, and this may well help here.

Second, appraisal can become a cosy chat, lacking challenge or focus. There can be collusion between the appraiser and appraisee. The supportive and formative element can become a bit too supportive. The GMC's specific supporting information requirements should ensure that at least decent evidence is considered at the appraisal. If the meeting allows rapport to be generated between appraiser and appraisee then that it is a welcome byproduct. (As an appraiser, I have always come away from appraisal interviews liking the appraisee more than before I started.)

Third, appraisal is very poor at detecting poor performance[11] (and medical appraisal is not actually designed to achieve detection of poor performance). In other industries appraisal is very much a performance review, against criteria, but in medicine appraisal is at best partially effective at this. Appraisal is good at providing positive evidence that some sort of CPD process is being followed, and the assumption is that if a doctor is pursuing CPD then they are showing conscientious concern about their performance. The inference is that a doctor who neglects their CPD is a poor one. However, most medical directors say that they become aware of poorly performing doctors through routes other than appraisal.[11] To a large extent, appraisal is the nice bit of the local clinical governance processes – the bit that confirms to the medical director that people are doing the right things.

Despite its limitations, appraisal is the best process we have developed so far for ensuring ongoing CPD and support for doctors by doctors. It is an opportunity, and it is worth making as much of this opportunity as you can.

References

1 Adams D. *The Hitch Hiker's Guide to the Galaxy*. London: Pan; 2009. If I were writing an entry about revalidation in this guide, I would probably put, 'Harmless (mostly)'.

2 Davies P, Walsh M, Pollock C. Performance management, appraisals, and revalidation: quantity analysis and quality control for UK GPs. *Br J Gen Pract*. 2011; **61**(589): 526–7.

3 Bennet G. *The Wound and the Doctor*. London: Secker & Warburg; 1987.

4 Riddell M. The *New Statesman* interview: Robert Winston. *New*

Statesman. 2000. Available at: www.newstatesman.com/node/136609 (accessed 15 December 2012).

5   Dalrymple T. A doctor's farewell. *Spectator*. 2005. Available at: www. spectator.co.uk/spectator/thisweek/13125/a-doctors-farewell.thtml (accessed 3 December 2012).

6   Tallis R. *Hippocratic Oaths: medicine and its discontents*. London: Atlantic Press; 2005.

7   General Medical Council. *Ready for Revalidation: making revalidation recommendations: the GMC responsible officer protocol*. London: General Medical Council; 2012. Available at: www.gmc-uk.org/static/documents/content/Responsible_Officer_Protocol.pdf (accessed 30 November 2012).

8   Coens T, Jenkins M. *Abolishing Performance Appraisals: why they backfire and what to do instead*. San Francisco: Berrett-Koehler; 2002.

9   McKinstry B, Evans A. Self assessment or self delusion. *Educ Primary Care*. 2006; **17**: 432–5.

10 Kruger J, Dunning D. Unskilled and unaware of it: how difficulties in recognizing one's own incompetence lead to inflated self-assessments. *J Pers Soc Psychol*. 1999; **77**(6): 1121–34.

11 Cox SJ, Holden JD. Presentation and outcome of clinical poor performance in one health district over a 5-year period: 2002–2007. *Br J Gen Pract*. 2009; **59**(562): 344–8.

Further reading

- Eve R. *PUNs and DENs: discovering learning needs in general practice*. Oxford: Radcliffe Publishing; 2003.
- Goldsmith M. *What Got You Here Won't Get You There: how successful people become even more successful*. London: Profile Books; 2008.
- Haynes K, Thomas M. *Clinical Risk Management in Primary Care*. Oxford: Radcliffe Publishing; 2005.
- National Patient Safety Agency. *Significant Event Audit*. London: NPSA; 2008. Available at: www.nrls.npsa.nhs.uk/resources/?entryid45=61500 (accessed 3 December 2012).
- Schön D. *The Reflective Practitioner: how professionals think in action*. Aldershot: Ashgate Publishing; 1991.
- Schulz K. *Being Wrong: adventures in the margin of error*. London: Portobello Books; 2010.
- Senge P. *The Fifth Discipline: the art and practice of the learning organisation*. London: Century Business; 1990.
- Vincent C. *Patient Safety*. 2nd ed. Chichester: Wiley-Blackwell; 2010.

Chapter 8

Personal development plans

Your decisions about your CPD activity at appraisal are usually crystallised by creating and maintaining a personal development plan (PDP). The appraiser will review progress under the revalidation headings and against the previous year's PDP goals. This progress is documented as part of the appraisal summary document

There is an art to setting PDP goals. They need to be interesting enough to be worth doing but not so large that they are unattainable. Some doctors need tiny, baby-step goals and some are only interested when the goals are large enough to be interesting. For example, if I had told my appraiser last year that I was going to write this book, he would have said, 'That's a huge goal, Peter. Shouldn't you break it up into smaller steps?'. Actually I have just finished one and now got onto this one, and it's nowhere on my PDPs at all! At some stage I will have to drag myself back to my PDP but it feels like duty, not interest, to me.

Personal development plan goals are supposed to be SMART – that is, specific, measurable, achievable, realistic and time-bound. Sometimes the goals are set as small, miserable, average, all too realistic and timid; sometimes they are stupendous, magnificent, awesome, revelatory and tremendous. For most doctors, keeping them somewhere between the extremes is sensible. There is a lot to be said for making them achievable, even though I suspect they then lack much stretch or stimulus for many appraisees. Jennings reviews this area thoroughly, and questions how well PDP goals match how we work out what we actually need to learn.[1]

Ideally, PDP goals are suggested by the doctor being appraised and confirmed and refined with the appraiser. As an appraiser, there is nothing worse than encountering an appraisee who makes no positive suggestions and expects you to come up with a ready-made plan for them. This results in irrelevant, boring PDP goals that are often ignored.

The number of PDP goals required is variable, depending on the doctor and their identified educational needs. The usual recommendation is between three and six goals. Ideally, the goals should be personal. Sometimes a doctor has a goal that is actually a project they can only complete by involving the whole practice – for example, to construct a practice business plan or a departmental development plan. It is not clear if this should count as a personal or a practice development goal.

Goals that involve many people, conversations and meetings are intrinsically harder to achieve but they may actually be what is needed at practice or departmental level. As yet, there is no system of practice development and practice appraisal. However, as an appraiser, I often feel that what I am seeing in one doctor's folder is an issue that needs to go to the whole practice team, but I can only deal with the individual doctor … and there is a tension here.

For appraisal PDP goals, keeping them within your own sphere of action and influence is more sensible, on the whole. Also, remember that, in terms of Stephen Covey's model of spheres of action,[2] the more effective you are within your sphere of action, the greater becomes your sphere of influence, and so the greater your eventual impact on your sphere of concern.

References

1   Jennings SF. Personal development plans and self-directed learning for healthcare professionals: are they evidence based? *Postgrad Med J.* 2007; **83**(982): 518–24.
2   Covey S. *The 7 Habits of Highly Effective People*. New York: Simon & Schuster; 2002.

Section 2

The evidence you need to produce for revalidation

Chapter 9

The General Medical Council's requirements for revalidation evidence

In March 2012, the GMC helpfully issued some clear guidance on the evidence it believes is relevant in appraisals. This guidance is referred to and quoted often throughout this book. The GMC is the statutory body for revalidation so if you are in any doubt about whose guidance to follow, the GMC's words usually have the lead.

The full GMC guidance is found here: www.gmc-uk.org/static/documents/content/Supporting_information_for_appraisal_and_revalidation.pdf (accessed 3 December 2012).

The GMC's six headings are

1 continuing professional development

2 quality improvement activity

3 significant events

4 feedback from colleagues

5 feedback from patients

6 review of complaints and compliments.

We discuss what is needed under each heading in the next few chapters.

For the five-year revalidation cycle, the requirements are about 50 hours of CPD per activity per year, including evidence of purposeful learning and reflection, in response to identified personal or service development needs. The activity needs to be logged, with evidence of time spent and reflections and learning points taken. The GMC does not set a specific target in terms of hours but following the suggestions from the medical Royal Colleges, about 50 hours seems to be a reasonable measure of 'enough'.

The quality improvement activity needs to be done once every five years. What counts as a quality improvement activity is quite wide, and the GMC guidance allows a certain amount of latitude here.

For significant events, you need to provide evidence of two per year, or 10 over five years. Multiple source feedback (MSF) and patient source feedback (PSF) need to be done once in five years. Review of complaints and compliments needs to be done each year at appraisal.

As long as the evidence of these activities is in your revalidation folder and appraisal summaries then the RO has enough evidence to work on.

You can do, and most doctors are already doing, far more than the minimum stated above. What you do need to understand is how to take what you are already doing and make sure it meets the requirements above. This may mean that you have to alter how you record and present your CPD rather than change what you actually are doing.

Revalidation is a slightly pedantic process and there is an element of the driving test and 'mirror, signal, manoeuvre' about it. For revalidation, the mirror may be the appropriate tool and the motto becomes, 'Yes sir. Look, I am reflecting now'. Perhaps we could summarise it as 'evidence, reflection, action' or 'as it is, as it should be, as it will be'.

It will in time be possible to become unreflectively reflective – for appraisal and revalidation purposes, the process of completing a structured reflective template may well be counted as good evidence of reflection – but for those of us who are naturally reflective such processes seem more constraining than real thought and reflection. They take a fluid and interesting process and turn it into a solid and rather boring piece of evidence. Our thoughts had already moved on and stopping to complete the recording process is a distraction, a bit like a 30 mph speed limit on a clear motorway.

We may need to accept that revalidation sets a rather minimal standard, and this is a bit like the teacher's lament that every once in a while they just about got their pupils to think (or at least look as if they were thinking).

Preliminary information for appraisal and revalidation

There are some preliminaries to the GMC evidence requirements which we need to comment on here.

First, you need correct demographic information for your appraiser. Then you must have a complete description of your scope of work – your main job, and any other subtitles and roles you have picked up. You must have the summary from the previous year's appraisals. You must have your PDP from the previous year. You must make a statement about probity and that yours is intact. You must make a health declaration.

These requirements can seem like mere formalities, and indeed mostly they are. However, there are some pitfalls to be wary of.

First, you do need to be acknowledging continuing development and achieving your PDP goals, or modifying them for sensible reasons. Simply ignoring them will raise unwanted questions about whether you are engaging with the process. Over time, your CPD activity should cover the needs of all your roles, not be skewed to just one particular special interest.

Second, the probity declaration is straightforward but if it is wrong or later comes under challenge, it could be reviewed. If you have a concern that your probity is under challenge, make sure the problem is acknowledged and reviewed at your appraisal. The danger of not so doing is that if you later come under challenge, the declaration comes to be seen as false and it shows that you lack insight into the problem and have not acted to manage the risk. In disciplinary scenarios such conclusions are not favourable for you.

Third, the health declaration. This is usually straightforward but it is important to make it accurately. The GMC is not particularly interested in your state of health. It is interested if you have a condition that poses a risk to your ability to do your job safely for patients. Its guidance states:

'A statement of health is a declaration that you accept the professional obligations placed on you in *Good Medical Practice* about your personal health'.

Good Medical Practice provides the following guidance.

'*Registration with a GP* – You should be registered with a general practitioner outside your family to ensure that you have access to independent and objective medical care. You should not treat yourself. (Paragraph 77)

Immunisation – You should protect your patients, your colleagues and yourself by being immunised against common serious communicable diseases where vaccines are available. (Paragraph 78)

A serious condition that could pose a risk to patients – If you know that you have, or think you might have, a serious condition that you could pass on to patients, of if your judgement or performance could be affected by a condition or its treatment, you must consult a suitably qualified colleague. You must ask for and follow their advice about investigations, treatment and changes to your practice that they consider necessary. You must not rely on your own assessment of the risk you pose to patients. (Paragraph 79)'

The problem from the GMC's viewpoint is the doctor who makes a mistake and ends up before a GMC (now Medical Practitioner Tribunal Service) panel. The illness is then produced as a defence or mitigation of the charge. The key question for the GMC is 'has the illness been acknowledged and managed sensibly to help the doctor get better and reduce any risk to patients?'.

If the health declaration has been completed honestly and accurately and there is evidence that the illness has been acknowledged and managed then the doctor has good insight and has acted sensibly for their own health and to protect patient safety. It is unlikely that the doctor would even come to GMC attention.

If, however, a doctor has for many years been making health declarations that 'everything's fine' and then it turns out that everything is not fine and that there is a significant medical problem which has not been acknowledged and which poses a risk to patient safety, then the GMC has evidence of 'lack of insight' and 'failure to protect patients from harm', both of which are liable to lead to disciplinary action against the doctor.

If you are a doctor with an illness then make sure you get treated properly by a colleague. This advice is for your own benefit – you are as entitled to decent treatment as anyone else – and to prevent the illness affecting your performance at work and so harming patients. As in first aid, the first casualty is ill but must not be allowed to create further casualties. Your own illness is a personal problem but if it affects your ability to provide safe medical care to patients then it needs managing as a clinical risk to others as well.

You do have an obligation to maintain yourself in a fit enough state of health to be able to perform your work, and not acknowledging this is risky behaviour.

Further information about doctors' health issues is provided in Appendix 1.

Chapter 10

Quality improvement activity

You are probably already doing a lot of this. You probably think about the quality of service you provide, are aware of gaps in quality and have already taken steps to do something about them. If, like most professionals, you are somewhat self-critical and often a bit of a perfectionist, then gaps in quality of service, whether due to your own ignorance or a system flaw, will annoy you. And when you experience this kind of problem you will probably want to improve the situation and get very frustrated if you cannot do something about it.

This section of the guidance aims to capture some evidence of these processes in action in you.

The GMC's guidance recommends:

'2. *Quality improvement activity*
For the purposes of revalidation, you will have to demonstrate that you regularly participate in activities that review and evaluate the quality of your work.

Quality improvement activities should be robust, systematic and relevant to your work. They should include an element of evaluation and action, and where possible, demonstrate an outcome or change.

Quality improvement activities could take many forms depending on the role you undertake and the work that you do. If you work in a non-clinical environment, you should participate in quality improvement activities relevant to your work. Examples of quality improvement activities include:

(i)   Clinical audit – evidence of effective participation in clinical audit or an equivalent quality improvement exercise that measures the care with which an individual doctor has been directly involved

(ii) Review of clinical outcomes – where robust, attributable and validated data are available. This could include morbidity and mortality statistics or complication rates where these are routinely recorded for local or national reports

(iii) Case review or discussion – a documented account of interesting or challenging cases that a doctor has discussed with a peer, another specialist or within a multidisciplinary team

(iv) Audit and monitor the effectiveness of a teaching programme

(v) Evaluate the impact and effectiveness of a piece of health policy or management practice.

If you work in a non-clinical role you might find it helpful to discuss options for a quality improvement activity with your appraiser, or a relevant professional association.'

As you can see here, the types of examples that count as relevant evidence in this section are wide, and give us latitude to show how we as individuals are committed to improving the quality of our work. This is a reasonable requirement on us as doctors. I believe that as doctors we are all committed to the quality of our work and to improving it. We all want to do better this year than last year. None of us is coming to work to deliberately do a bad job.

Bringing this intrinsic drive for quality of professionals into the open, and checking that we are contributing and doing it well is actually a positive thing. Reviewing our work at appraisal with an experienced colleague can help us improve our performance and effectiveness. Why would we not want to be doing something like this?

So for revalidation, we need to demonstrate some area in which we have acted to monitor and improve the quality of our work. We probably are doing this a lot of the time. For revalidation, you need one good example of this from the last five years. The example you choose should be personal to you, and something on which you have led.

It is up to you to choose your example but the GMC's instructions above allow a wide range of activity to be counted as quality improvement activity. Even as a peripatetic locum, you will still have a deep personal and professional concern about the quality of your work, and how you improve it. At the very least, you will have a few good cases from which a case discussion can emerge.

The key components of a quality improvement activity are:

- identification of a problem – a flaw or gap in quality
- definition and understanding of the problem
- consideration of the problem in light of the experience of others, e.g. in the literature, in professional guidance
- action taken to improve the problem
- outcomes seen as the result of this action
- plans for further improvements, maintenance of existing improvements.

In short, the quality improvement activity shows evidence of reflection in action, and of you as an individual doctor thinking about your work and taking clear action to improve it.

Thinking from a patient viewpoint, you would want to be treated by a doctor involved in some reflection like this. You would want a doctor who reflected on their work and was not simply satisfied to do what had always been done before, or one who simply accepted the flaws in the system as 'just the way it is around here'. You would not want an unreflective doctor who just 'works here'. You would want an engaged and active doctor who thinks about their work and is acting to improve it.

And actually most doctors I have met want to improve the quality of their work and enjoy discussing their plans to achieve it. What frustrates doctors is when there is a clear problem but they are unable to mobilise enough support to achieve the improvement necessary. At this point, the gap between the clinical need and the system's offering to that need can seem vast and insuperable and can be experienced as stress in the individual doctor. If we improve our ability at quality improvement we may reduce our stress and instead find ourselves sorting out a manageable problem, which is rewarding and interesting.

The positive intention behind the quality improvement activity is to show that we as individual doctors do care about the quality of our work and service provision, and that we actively do something about this.

Following on from this, it becomes apparent that:

- quality improvement is a concern of every doctor
- we may not all be effective at achieving this (but at least we try)

- there is a need for doctors to learn about how best to achieve and implement quality improvement in their work

- achieving quality improvement of individuals and services is the key role of clinical leadership so all doctors must be involved at some level in clinical leadership.

This part of the revalidation process can be seen as leading us into accepting our role in clinical leadership. Clinical leadership can be seen as the creative transformation of glitches and problems into free-flowing systems of care for patients.

Chapter 11

Significant event audit

The GMC guidance (emphasis mine) here is:

'Significant events
A significant event (also known as an untoward or critical incident) is *any unintended or unexpected event, which could or did lead to harm of one or more patients.* This includes incidents which did not cause harm but could have done, or where the event should have been prevented. These events should be collected routinely by your employer, where you are directly employed by an organisation, and hospitals should have formal processes in place for logging and responding to all events. If you are self-employed, you should make note of any such events or incidents and undertake a review.'

It goes on to recommend that at appraisal the discussion should include:

'Participation – As a doctor you have a responsibility to log incidents and events according to the reporting process within your organisation. Discussion at appraisal should include your participation in logging any incidents or events and your participation in any clinical governance meetings where incidents or events and learning are discussed.

Lessons learnt – You should be able to demonstrate that you are aware of any patterns in the types of incidents or events recorded about your practice and discuss any lessons learnt. Discussion at appraisal should include any systematic learning from errors and events such as investigations and analysis, and the development of solutions and implementation of improvements. Areas for further learning and development should be reflected in your personal development plan and CPD.

Take action – Your appraiser will be interested in any actions you took or any changes you implemented to prevent such events or incidents happening again.'

As in all the evidence for revalidation, the emphasis is on identifying problems, reflecting and learning from them, and then taking action to mitigate the risks. Such behaviour is a basic part of any professional's practice and it is obvious why it is in the portfolio of evidence requested for revalidation. A doctor not responding to SEAs and not looking to mitigate risks would be a danger to their patients.

It is worth noting the GMC definition of significant events here. The criteria of potential or actual harm and actions taken in review and to prevent recurrence shape this activity. It goes a long way beyond just reviewing a case.

The terms significant event analysis (SEA), serious untoward incident (SUI) and critical incident reporting (CIR) are not entirely clear or exclusive, nor are they exact synonyms. The definitions of 'serious' , 'significant' and 'critical' are not completely circumscribed and so what one doctor thinks is an SEA may be a minor glitch to another. The terms are not used consistently across the NHS. For revalidation, it is important that any incident that raises a major risk to patient safety is reviewed and learned from, rather than what it is called. The GMC's definition of an SEA as 'any unintended or unexpected event, which could or did lead to harm of one or more patients' gives a clear pointer to what sort of events should be included in this section. All events under this rubric should be analysed and included in your appraisals.

Some College guidelines, such as the Royal College of General Practitioners', recommend that you need two SEAs per year (or 10 over five years). This is a helpful guide to the amount required but not actually what the GMC is asking for, which is that all SEAs (using its definition) should be reviewed. I think the hardest part with SEAs is not finding enough but the risk of finding too many. You do not have to be in a surgery long before you realise that every consultation is risky! Every consultation has within it some potential for error. We hope we know enough to avoid these errors but experience shows that even with well-intentioned doctors and much past summarised information and many computer-generated alerts, errors still happen.

What is amazing about medical practice is not how often errors occur but how often they are avoided, partly by professional diligence, partly by good computer and other systems, and partly by luck. The feeling that there are many 'great saves' and 'narrow misses' each day is huge.

Significant events are important because they show that you are aware of what is going on in and around your work, you notice what is wrong, or potentially could go wrong, and take action to mitigate such risks. The biggest danger here is not the doctor who has lots of incidents happening around them but the one who is ignoring them and never reporting or noticing any. You could probably make a system-wide case to provide incentives for reporting SEAs, on the grounds that encouraging SEAs could reduce later problems from more severe events such as negligence claims.

Significant events remind us of risks in our practice and of the importance of doing something to reduce those risks. This is sensible clinical and managerial practice and done consistently over time, it will tend to reduce risks to patients. It also helps us to be accountable amongst and to our colleagues, and to help keep our vigilance up.

When writing up SEAs, the following guidance from the RCGP guide to revalidation (www.rcgp.org.uk/revalidation-and-cpd/revalidation-guidance-for-gps.aspxis) provides a useful structure.

'An account of a significant event audit should not allow patients to be identified and should comprise:

- the title of the event

- the date of the event

- the date the event was discussed and the roles of those present

- a description of the event involving the GP

- what went well

- what could have been done differently

- reflections on the event in terms of:

  - knowledge, skills and performance

  - safety and quality

  - communication, partnership and teamwork

  - maintaining trust

51

- what changes have been agreed:
  - for me personally
  - for the team
- changes carried out and their effect.'

Chapter 12

Continuing professional development

The GMC's instructions here are:

'1. *Continuing professional development*
Continuing professional development (CPD) is a continuous learning process that complements formal undergraduate and postgraduate education and training in order to maintain and further develop competence and performance. CPD enables you to maintain and improve across all areas of your practice.

Good Medical Practice requires you to keep your knowledge and skills up to date and encourages you to "take part in educational activities that maintain and further develop" your competence and performance. (Paragraph 12) CPD should encourage and support specific changes in practice and career development and be relevant to your practice. CPD is not an end in itself.

By its nature, CPD must be tailored to the specific needs and interests of you and your practice. There are numerous ways that you could demonstrate your CPD. Participation in a College or Faculty run CPD scheme will be one way of demonstrating that you are keeping up to date in relation to your practice. Further guidance is available from the individual Colleges and Faculties. The GMC does not require doctors to participate in College or Faculty run CPD schemes.

Frequency: There should be a discussion on CPD at each appraisal meeting.'

You will see from this that there is a requirement for CPD but no great specificity about what has to be done, or how much. This is both an opportunity for us as doctors and a problem. This leads us to some questions which I will try to answer clearly.

What is continuing professional development?

Continuing professional development is educational activity directed towards a specific professional learning need. It is focused on answering specific questions that have arisen in your professional work. Or that will arise as you try to improve your work next year. Or implement a new process or operation.

The GMC wants our CPD to be focused on outcomes rather than inputs such as hours spent or credits earned. It is more interested in why the CPD is being done than in how long it takes you to do it.

So the aim in CPD is to show the following.

- Why did I do this piece of CPD?

- What question did it answer for me?

- What need in me or a patient did it meet?

- Why this method of learning?

- What will the outcome be as a result of the new learning?

- What have I learned from it?

- What will improve for patients?

- What will improve for the local NHS system?

The Royal Colleges recommend some anchoring of CPD in time, suggesting that 50 hours of CPD activity per year is a sensible minimum. The argument is that at least time is measurable whereas showing definite learning and improved outcomes from learning is not always easy.

The battle here is between those who think CPD needs to be measurable and recordable and those for whom the real benefit of CPD is the thought and reflection it opens up. I agree more with the latter view but the practical side of me says at least if 50 hours is specified, it can to some extent be recorded and measured. The risk of measuring hours is that a competition develops to score the most hours of CPD, whereas the person who has learned one thing well that year may actually have achieved more than all the recorded hyperactive CPD of their colleague.

What you need to show for continuing professional development

The basic requirement is for some sort of learning log that records what CPD you undertake and what you learn from it. The suggested headings might be as follows.

- Date of event
- Title
- Why was this piece of CPD needed? State the clinical or educational need it addresses
- Time spent on event (to nearest hour)
- What was done?
- What was the outcome from this event? For me? For patients? For anyone else?
- What key learning points do I take from this event?
- What is the next action I need to make as a result of this?

The aim is to show at least 50 hours of educational activity each year, which is purposeful and which meets your own specific educational needs. As in all the revalidation guidance, the aim is to show identification of learning needs/gaps in service, and that you recognise these and take steps to meet them. The process is a classic example of Donald Schön's great process of 'reflection in action'.

For most of us, recording between 50 and 100 hours of CPD activity per year, which is done properly and reflected and acted upon, is plenty and more than meets the requirements of revalidation.

The CPD log is reviewed at appraisal and the claim for hours/credits is verified by your appraiser. The RO will take the appraiser's verification as accurate.

In most specialties, one hour of CPD activity is counted as one credit. For GPs, the RCGP recommends that if an activity can be shown to have had significant impact beyond the individual doctor then one hour of activity can be counted as two credits.

You will note that the GMC has not recommended any specific amounts of activity for CPD, preferring to focus activity towards outcomes rather than measure inputs.

Responsible officers need to know that you have CPD processes in place and are actively using them and learning through them. Given the GMC guidance, they are unlikely to be bothered about a few hours or credits either side of a rather arbitrary target. But if there is a lack of CPD activity they, and their appraisers, will be concerned about you.

How should I record my continuing professional development activity?

You can record your CPD activity in any way you like – paper based, spreadsheet, electronic, toolkit. The key requirements are that it is happening and that you can show reflection, learning, outcomes and actions coming from it.

What your appraiser and RO are really looking for is not the details of what you have done but that CPD is happening and is purposeful and reflective. Provided your log confirms this then it achieves what is needed.

What counts as continuing professional development?

The range of activities recognised for CPD is wide. It can include practically any occasion on which clinical learning is happening. The basic checklist of events that can count includes:

- courses
- lectures and seminars
- team meetings and reviews (educational, rather than business meetings)
- educational group discussions
- time spent on audit
- time spent on preparation, e.g. of teaching, of an article
- personal reading where it meets a clinical educational goal
- online modules on specific topics.

The key requirement for appraisal and revalidation is that learning is focused around an identified clinical or managerial need, and leads to reflection and new learning and action. If your learning can be shown to do this then it will count as CPD.

Chapter 13

Multiple source (colleague) feedback

'O wad some Pow'r the giftie gie us
To see oursels as others see us
It wad frae monie a blunder free us
An' foolish notion
What airs in dress an' gait wad lea'e us
An' ev'n Devotion.' (Burns, *To a Louse*)

Burns' verse translates into modern English as:

'Oh, that God would give us the smallest of gifts
To be able to see ourselves as others see us
It would save us from many mistakes
and foolish thoughts
We would change the way we look and gesture
and to how and what we apply our time and attention.'

Colleague feedback (also known as multiple source feedback (MSF) or 360° feedback) gives us the opportunity to do this. It answers the question, 'How do I come across to others?'. Gaining such insight is both fascinating and frightening.

It is the part of the revalidation evidence that is potentially the most useful in generating insight and also potentially the part with the biggest risk of problems. Even at a gathering of senior doctors (ROs, MDs and appraisal leads), there was much concern about this aspect of revalidation. It was interesting that we were much more scared of our colleagues' view of us than of our patients' feedback.

In this chapter I hope to allay these worries and suggest sensible ways to give and receive such feedback. There is a lot to learn from our colleagues and we want to get something useful out of all this. Or at least enough to get through revalidation intact.

The evidence we have suggests that we only partially know ourselves and our strengths and weaknesses.[1] To get a fuller picture of our effectiveness, we need the help of others to see both our strengths and weaknesses, so we can play to or mitigate these and be more effective.[2]

We are all going to be both giving and receiving this feedback and so we need to think about how we can do this well for each other.

The Johari Window

The classic model here is the Johari Window.[3] This proposes that we have four quadrants within which we operate.

The first is the public arena – what I know about me, and what you know about me. In this arena information is largely public and shared.

The second quadrant is our blind spots – the other knows something about me that I do not know or recognise myself. Colleague and patient feedback may help us to see our blind spots, and we may or may not like what we see. But we are probably going to be better if we can face such feedback, reflect on it, and learn something from it. It may at times be uncomfortable but perhaps we should remember what the poet Rilke wrote about responding to challenges.[4]

'Winning does not tempt that man.
This is how he grows: by being defeated, decisively,
by constantly greater beings.'

Perhaps we need to acknowledge some greater beings amongst our colleagues and patients? Perhaps the humility to acknowledge this is the greatest strength of all.

The third quadrant is our facade – I know some things about myself but others do not know them. We spend a fair amount of effort on maintaining our facades and hoping no-one sees through them but I suspect that others may know more about us than we realise. If we are lucky, they will see what we are doing with some compassion. (Remember they may be maintaining their own facades just as actively as we maintain our own.) If we are unlucky, the others may puncture our facade and there may be some risk and some discomfort here.

The final quadrant is the unknown shadow area of life – there's something neither you nor I know about myself. If you like a Jungian approach, in this area there are major opportunities for development, many hidden talents and also some of our deepest fears. This combination of discovery and fear is why many avoid visting here.[5]

In colleague and patient feedback we may gather, or be forced into, insights across all four quadrants of the Johari Window, and have to deal with the resultant learning that emerges.

The next part of this chapter outlines a method of doing this in a benign and helpful way, which I hope will help colleagues to do this sort of feedback well, effectively and safely.

Giving multiple source feedback for a colleague

Remember that the point of giving this feedback is to help your colleague improve. You may want to settle scores or bury the hatchet in your colleague. You may want to tell them exactly what for, and why, and you may have some well-justified reasons for wanting to do so. But may I suggest that you bury the hatchet in the garden, take a breath and then think about suggestions to help your colleague improve?

First, you still have to work with the colleague and if they recognise your animosity then things will be worse afterwards.

Second, you are giving feedback, not setting yourself up as judge and jury over your colleague.

Third, remember that the measure you give will be the measure you receive, and that you will always fear the one you have attacked. And you have yet to get your own MSF results.

Fourth, remember to describe your colleague's good points; they will have many of these so give credit where it is due. You don't become a decent doctor by accident but by deliberate, purposeful learning and practice.[6,7] Recognise this, and if you know your colleague's background well, acknowledge the cost they have paid to gain it.

Fifth, try to describe your colleague's flaws and weaknesses as behaviours rather than character or existential problems. You do want to nudge them[8] towards improvements but you can help by presenting the nudge in such a way as to gain co-operation rather than opposition. You are helping to frame their 'choice architecture', as Sunstein and Thaler describe it.[8] Earlier praise and understanding (as above) can help build some rapport before delivering a message 'but could be better still if ...'. If the 'but' appears too soon or too sharply, it will simply invalidate what has gone before. Remember that your colleague would already have done something about their flaws if they knew about them. Your job is to gently reveal them to your colleague. And remember that what we criticise and recognise in others often applies with some force to ourselves too. This does not invalidate your feedback but it does leave you vulnerable to a 'Tu quoque' response.

Sixth, if you are marking your colleague very low on a clinical attribute, do you really have a performance concern about your colleague? If so, do not leave it to the feedback form. As the recent GMC guidance makes clear, you have a duty to act if you are concerned that a colleague's poor performance puts patients at risk. If you are at that level of concern, speak to the medical director directly and leave the MSF questionnaire unanswered.

It is better to give feedback as constructive suggestions for improvement. Consider the three questions that the doctor seeking feedback is really looking to answer.

- What do I do well?
- What would you like me to do more of?
- What would you like me to do less of?

When approached in this frame of reference, you can give fair feedback, with the positive intention of helping your colleague to do better in the future. This frame of reference makes the whole process safer for both the giver and recipient of feedback, and increases the chances of successful behaviour change by the recipient.

Advice about receiving multiple source feedback

Marshall Goldsmith has written a good book on MSF with the great title of *What Got You Here Won't Get You There*.[2] Goldsmith's key point is that most of us have got to where we are partially because of who we are and our great knowledge and talents and partially because other people have been kind enough to ignore or work around our ignorance, foibles and unpleasant idiosyncrasies. Perhaps with PSF and MSF we will be able to develop our good points further and in turn knock some of the rough edges off our bad points.

Goldsmith mainly works with senior managers at the level just below senior directors, and those who may be the next people to come through as senior directors. At the lower levels, and hidden within an organisation, these people's idiosyncrasies may be tolerable but once they are in an exposed position as a chief executive officer or similar, their foibles could become major issues that could threaten the viability of their organisations. In our work as doctors, we are moving ever more into leadership roles such as commissioning, so getting used to PSF and MSF will become a necessary step in every doctor's development.

When receiving feedback, we need to be both resilient and sensitive. We need to pick up the consistent signals about what needs to improve. We need not to be too sensitive to critical comments, and to accept that they are offered positively as a stimulus to improvement, rather than as an attack on our character. We need to be a bit careful about who we ask to offer MSF to us before sending the questionnaires round. But we also need to remember that whether you ask people who you think like you or people who you think do not like you, the results of MSF tend to be same. If there is a consistent trend indicating that you need to change something, both your friends and your enemies will let you know.

Remember that the GMC's MSF form[9] is fairly mundane; it asks very basic clinical questions and simple questions about interactions with colleagues. It is very much focused on the here and now of medical practice. So the information you get will be useful if you are working in medical practice, rather than in management settings.

Outlying responses can be discarded as they probably do not fully reflect the reality of your work. However, if responses are all trending in a certain direction then the pattern becomes noteworthy, and your reflection on the feedback should be that it has been noted.

What the GMC is looking for here[10] is:

> *'Discussing colleague feedback and patient feedback at your appraisal*
> *Respond to the questionnaire feedback* – You should receive your questionnaire feedback prior to your appraisal to ensure you have had time to consider it and are prepared to discuss it. You should be able to demonstrate that you have reflected on the feedback. Your appraiser will be interested in what actions you took as a result of the feedback, not just that you collected it.
> *Identify opportunities for professional development and improvement* – The discussion at appraisal should highlight areas of good performance and help you to identify any areas that might require further development. This should be reflected in your

61

personal development plan and your choices for continuing professional development.

Cover your whole practice – The exercise should reflect the whole scope of your practice. The range of patients providing feedback should reflect the range of patients that you see. The selection of colleagues will depend on the nature of your practice. We recommend that you ask as wide a range of colleagues as possible and this might include colleagues from other specialties, junior doctors, nurses, allied healthcare professionals, and management and clerical staff.

Doctors that do not see patients, or cannot collect feedback from their patients – One of the principles of revalidation is that patient feedback should be at the heart of doctors' professional development. You should assume that you do have to collect patient feedback, and consider how you can do so. We recommend that you think broadly about who can give you this sort of feedback. For instance, you might want to collect views from people who are not conventional patients but have a similar role, like families and carers, students, or even suppliers or customers.

We recognize that, due to the nature of particular types of practice, it may not be appropriate for some doctors to collect feedback from their patients. If you believe that you cannot collect feedback from your patients, you should discuss this (as well as any alternative ways to engage with your patients) with your appraiser.

Number of respondents required – The GMC is not prescribing the number of colleague and patient responses you are required to collect. We recommend that you check with your employer or questionnaire provider, as each questionnaire will have been piloted to determine the appropriate number of respondents required to provide an accurate picture of your practice. If you are using the GMC questionnaires, we have guidance available online. In any event, it is in your best interests to have as many completed responses as possible to ensure the feedback reflects the totality of your work.'

What you need to do

1 Gather the MSF from colleagues.

2 Use the forms available on the GMC website (or another format which asks the relevant questions about you personally and your

working habits; or your employer may have a specific system it provides for this).

3 Ask a neutral person, e.g. the practice manager, to collate responses for you.

4 Fill in the form yourself to see what your self-rating is.

5 Include responses from a wide range of colleagues. Colleagues here include direct departmental and practice colleagues, those senior and junior to you, people who take referrals from you, e.g. MAU team, A&E department, people to whom you supply information, e.g. consultants to GPs, nursing colleagues, pharmacy colleagues (they often know you very well), local managers, colleagues on bodies such as the LMC, commissioning groups, learned societies.

6 Reflect on the information received at your appraisal interview. In particular, does your view of yourself and your work and abilities match that of your colleague? If there is a mismatch, what are the reasons for this?

7 Record your results, your thoughts and reflections in an appropriate format, ready to present them to your appraiser.

In medicine we all know and interact with many others. The aim here is to find out what we do well and what we do not do so well, and learn about what we can do better in future.

The aim is to get at least 15 responses. Think widely about how many people know something about you – it will be a far bigger number than your direct colleagues. The more responses you receive the better. As far as can be told, somewhere between 15 and 30 responses on MSF is plenty to achieve a useful picture of how you come across to colleagues and what areas need improving.

The weaknesses of the current arrangements are that they are not fully electronic so paper is needed and then some laborious number crunching (you can get round this by paying for an electronic service or using a service such as Survey Monkey), and there is a lack of national comparison data on scores so you cannot easily see how you compare to others locally, nationally and in your specialty.

In time, MSF forms will be built into electronic formats and then will allow for electronic compilation and comparison with large numbers of others. I suspect that electronic versions of MSF will become available over the next 12 months but for now (autumn 2012) we are stuck with paper formats.

The General Medical Council's form

I have just (September 2012) completed my own MSF using the GMC's form. My impression of the form is that its questions are very clinically focused, with very little asking about our management abilities or our behaviour in meetings. It is fine as far as it goes for learning about how others see your direct clinical work, but offers very little insight about how you function in your wider context of work. I asked many managers I work with at the Commissioning Group for feedback, and many of the answers they gave could only be 'don't know'. The space for free-text comments on the form was small, and this discouraged people from writing much here.

Conclusion

The colleague feedback part of revalidation has potentially a lot of learning in it. I hope the guidance I have given here will help colleagues with giving and receiving such feedback. I hope we will all use it as a tool to encourage improvement in ourselves and our colleagues.

References

1   Halvorson HG. You are (probably) wrong about you. *Harvard Business Review.* htpps://blogs.hbr.org/cs/2012/07/you_are_probably_wrong_about_y.html (accessed 15 December 2012).

2   Goldsmith M. *What Got You Here Won't Get You There: how successful people become even more successful.* London: Profile Books; 2008.

3   Johari Window: http://psychcentral.com/blog/archives/2008/07/08/the-johari-window/ (accessed 16 December 2012).

4   Rilke RM. The Man Watching: www.poetry-chaikhana.com/R/RilkeRainerM/ManWatching.htm (accessed 16 December 2012).

5   Zweig C, Wolf S. *Romancing the Shadow: how to access the hidden power in our dark side.* London: Thorsons; 1997.

6   Colvin G. *Talent is Overrated: what really separates world-class performers from everybody else.* London: Nicholas Brealey; 2008.

7   Syed M. *Bounce: how champions are made.* London: Fourth Estate; 2010.

8   Sunstein C, Thaler R. *Nudge. Improving decisions about health, wealth and happiness.* London: Penguin: 2009.

9   General Medical Council: www.gmc-uk.org/static/documents/content/Developing_implementing_and_administering_questionnaires_.pdf (accessed 3 December 2012).

10 General Medical Council: www.gmc-uk.org/doctors/revalidation/colleague_patient_feedback_intro.asp (accessed 3 December 2012).

Chapter 14

Patient source feedback

This gives us the opportunity to answer the question, 'How do I come across to my patients?'. Ultimately revalidation is about giving a good service to patients. It makes sense to find out from your patients if you are achieving this.

What has been said above about colleague feedback also applies to gathering feedback from patients. Here the aim is to get feedback from most of the types of patients you meet. For GPs, this means covering a range of ages and characters. For a specialist, it would mean a good spread of the patients at their clinic. It is also worthwhile including some indirect patients – carers and relatives – in the sample.

It is reckoned for this feedback that about 35 responses are needed to get a decent sample size. That's about one day's worth of consultations for a GP.

As with colleague feedback, what you are looking for is trends and tendencies. Outlying scores are unlikely to be accurate and can probably be safely ignored.

The patients have had even less training on giving feedback than we have and so there will be some roughness in their comments. Patients may not know about medicine but they are often observant and have a fair idea about which doctors they like and dislike and why. They are often good at working out what's going on for a doctor, and whether they can give good advice and service or not. And at the end of the day, the patients are the ones who receive our ministrations and so they have more interest than most in encouraging good doctors to do well. The patient perspective on our work is a good one to include in revalidation. The process would be less convincing without it.

For revalidation, the requirement is to gather this feedback, reflect on it, see what you learn from it and what action you will take after it.

The GMC has a suitable form available on its website. If you use an alternative format, it needs to be based on good medical practice and ask questions about you personally as a doctor. The old practice or departmental survey is about the organisation, not about you as an individual.

The same drawbacks about colleague feedback and the information gathering and current paper forms apply to patient feedback. They will be remedied over forthcoming months but for those doing this in the next few months (March–December 2013), the difficulty of working with paper forms has to be accepted.

Having done my own patient feedback in September 2012, my impression is that the form is fair and asks the right questions about my performance, and what patients will notice about it. It was more useful for me than the colleague feedback.

Further reading

- General Medical Council. www.gmc-uk.org/doctors/revalidation/colleague_patient_feedback_intro.asp (accessed 3 December 2012).

Chapter 15

Response to concerns and complaints

We live in an audit society. Fortunately, we sometimes live in a plaudit society as well. Either is useful evidence in this section of your appraisal documentation.

What the appraiser (and behind them, the RO) is looking for here is that concerns and complaints are dealt with well and resolved sensibly, ideally with some learning along the way.

These days all doctors get some complaints each year. We none of us can entirely avoid them. We know that our first response to a complaint about us will not be 'Oh great, here's a golden opportunity for some learning' but rather along the lines of anger, irritation and sadness. We do tend to be upset by complaints.

However, once that initial emotional phase has passed by and you have had a cup of tea and settled down a bit then you get into the sorting out phase. And in this phase the art of crafting a careful reply to a complaint comes into play. Review and reflection on the case occur. Much discussion with medical defence organisation colleagues occurs. Some review with more experienced colleagues will be useful. The doctor and the team will work to develop a good response to the complaint. The process is not entirely enjoyable but there is a lot to be learned from it.

This part of the revalidation process is looking to see that complaints are dealt with well, if there are any trends or patterns and whether learning and altered behaviour are occurring as a result.

As the GMC guidance puts it:

'*Discussing complaints and compliments at your appraisal*

Awareness – You should be aware of the complaints procedures in the organisations you work in and be aware of any complaints received about you or your team.

Participation in the investigation and response – You should participate in the investigation and response to the complainant where appropriate. You should show that you are aware of the advice in *Good Medical Practice* when investigating and responding to complaints, and in the continued treatment of the complainant, where appropriate.

Actions taken in response to the complaint – Your appraiser will be interested in what actions you took as a result of the complaint and any modification in practice that has resulted, either individually or across the team.

Identify opportunities for professional development – Complaints may potentially act as an indicator of performance and the way in which you use your professional and clinical skills. Discussion at appraisal should highlight areas for further learning, which should then be included in your personal development plan and continuous professional development.'

What you need as evidence

- A list of complaints and compliments received (I suspect negligence actions and settlements should count as a form of complaint but at present there is no formal requirement to include these, which is a weakness in the current system).

- A brief summary of each complaint: include the main issue behind the complaint (leave names and patient-identifiable data out to comply with patient confidentiality – not 'Mrs Jones' but 'a 68-year-old woman ...'. You will remember who sent the complaint in, and the RO and appraiser just want to know that you handled the complaint well).

- Some evidence about how you responded appropriately and sensitively to the complaint.

- Some evidence that you have considered the issues raised by the complaints, learned from the experience, and if necessary made adaptations to your practice.

- Some evidence that you have looked to see if any overall patterns emerge from the complaints you have received.

In other words, complaints are seen as a form of feedback about our work. The question is, what can you learn from this feedback? Are the themes from the complaints mirrored elsewhere, for example in your patient or colleague feedback?

At appraisal

Formally the appraiser is looking to see that complaints have been dealt with sensitively and sensibly.

Complaints can be bruising experiences and leave emotional scars. One of the tasks an appraiser can sometimes usefully perform is to check that the doctor has recovered fully from the experience, and is not taking bad feeling forward into the next year. If you have had a complaint that has left bad feeling, by all means ask your appraiser to help with this or suggest further support you could access.

Of course, if you have fully dealt with the complaint and it is clearly in the past both for the patient and the doctor, then just describe the event for the appraisal records and do not go back to agonise over it again.

Compliments

Just as complaints need analysing, compliments also need recording and analysing. They too are great feedback. Enjoy them, and see what you can learn from them. At the very least, they allow us a nice break from complaints.

As humans, we tend to particularly notice what is wrong with things and comment about them. This is a useful ability; for example, it enhances a doctor's diagnostic ability. However, every so often it is worth noticing just how much is right with life and work, how much goes well, and showing appreciation for this. We tend to concentrate on small problems against a background of so much more that is right.

When people compliment us on what we are doing right, it is fair to celebrate this and enjoy the appreciation. Accept it with thanks.

Chapter 16

How should I present this evidence to my appraiser?

If any issue has made appraisal harder in the last few years, it is the withdrawal of support from the NHS appraisal toolkit. That toolkit was not perfect but most of us had got used to using it and its headings and were working to improve our presentation of data. The appraisers likewise were learning how to make their Form 4 summaries more complete and useful.

Anyway, the old toolkit was closed down on information governance grounds and the replacement product is not immediately obvious. Various colleges, organisations and commercial companies have offered toolkits but none is currently seen as the obvious answer to the problem. The current (December 2012) best option seems to be the MAG3 document on the Revalidation Support Team's website: www.revalidationsupport.nhs.uk/responsible_officer/responsible_ officer_mag.php. Many areas are recommending its use but of course a recommendation is not mandatory. You can present the evidence in another format but the MAG3 is the best document at present for this task.

For doctors being appraised, there are two fundamental tasks here: gathering the information and storing it securely, and displaying it well to make the appraiser's and RO's roles easy.

The MAG3 document facilitates the display of information. It is designed to make the appraisal interview easy to conduct. The output is designed to make the communication between appraiser and RO easy to achieve so that the RO is assured that the appraisal has happened, and that reasonable evidence has been presented and recorded.

Gathering the information needs to be done in any convenient format – probably word-processed documents for most things and maybe a spreadsheet for the learning log. You need to keep your raw material together in one place on your computer so that you know where it is.

For the MAG3 document, you need to integrate your raw materials into the MAG3 interactive pdf. You should present summary documents that collectively do not exceed 10 Mb of space. If you are going over the 10 Mb limit, you are probably showing too much raw material rather than focused descriptions of data and your reflections about them. Think again about what you are presenting to your appraiser – they do not need large raw data files or many pictures. It is very unlikely that you or they will want to go back into original data files for appraisal purposes. A brief note that they are available for inspection if needed is more than sufficient. Like you, your appraiser is not short of material to read.

In time, we may get a secure appraisal toolkit that is good at gathering evidence, prompting appropriate reflection, allowing easy access and interchange between appraiser and appraisee, and then sending appropriate outputs to the ROs. We do not have such a toolkit yet.

The ROs have an 'RO dashboard' that connects them to the GMC, through which they will send their revalidation recommendations to the GMC.

As the doctor being revalidated, you have already connected yourself to the GMC electronically, at GMC Online, haven't you? So you can get the good news about your revalidation quickly and easily? If not, go to this link: www.gmc-uk.org/doctors/information_for_doctors/gmc_online.asp.

Chapter 17

Sessional doctors and other atypical scenarios

Some patterns of work make gathering evidence for appraisal and revalidation harder than others. Some patterns of work are intrinsically more isolated and individualistic. Although medicine used to be a profession of rugged individualists, these days we are moving to a more collaborative and team-based approach, and probably this is mostly an improvement. Some isolated patterns of work, e.g. solo practitioners, out-of-hours doctors or peripatetic locums, are also more exposed to medico-legal risks. Patients have a right to expect that all doctors they encounter are fit to practise and up to date. Whatever your pattern of work, the requirements for revalidation and appraisal apply to us all as doctors equally, and so individual doctors need to find a way to meet them. This may be a direct method or by means of an 'equivalent portfolio' that meets the revalidation requirements.

The doctors who may come under 'non-standard' include the following.

- Those in clinical general practice who may find elements of a standard portfolio difficult to accumulate; this includes doctors whose main or only work is as:
  - peripatetic locums
  - out-of-hours doctors (and those working in similar clinical contexts such as in walk-in centres)
  - GPs in remote or very small practices
  - GPs in the defence medical services or the Foreign and Commonwealth Office
  - GPs working in secure environments.

- Those who were not in work for all years in the five-year revalidation cycle or who are on extended career breaks, including those working overseas.

- GP registrars whose licence becomes due for renewal (the deanery will manage this).

- Those whose only or predominant work as a doctor is not clinical but is in NHS management, educational management, political roles, health informatics, academia or staff appointments within the defence medical services (who may remain on the GMC Register but can let their licences to practise lapse).

The RCGP's guide to revalidation says:

'An equivalent portfolio is intended to reflect and to be more appropriate to the working environment of the doctor concerned. One key aspect for peripatetic locums and doctors who work in out-of-hours services or in walk-in centres is the frequent absence of organisational and peer group support. One solution is the development of mechanisms to reduce the professional isolation that many of these doctors experience. The models for this that have been identified include:

- general practices, federations and out-of-hours organisations that frequently employ GPs on short-term, sessional contracts must recognise their responsibility to all their employees, including these doctors. They should inform and involve doctors in any significant event or complaint that relates to them; they should facilitate access to the clinical records of patients treated by these doctors for the purposes of clinical audit and quality improvement; and they should support the conduct of patient surveys

- professional organisations that support the working lives and professional development of peripatetic locums are becoming more established. The National Association of Sessional GPs (www.nasgp.org.uk/) has developed the "chambers" model through which contracts, bookings, education and quality assurance are supported collectively by other locum doctors. Other organisations, such as the North East Locum Group (www.nelg.org.uk/), act as an information forum in a specific area, advertising local educational events, running educational meetings and providing space for locums and practices to advertise. The

General Practitioners Committee (GPC)'s Sessional GP subcommittee (http://bma.org.uk/about-the-bma/how-we-work/negotiating-committees/ general-practitioners-committee) is also able to offer valuable support

- educational groups (locum groups, self-directed learning groups, etc.) are also developing. In these, doctors working outside supportive organisations meet to share experience and learn together. Such educational groups may well be virtual if that works for the participants.

Although there are some circumstances in which such mechanisms are impractical, it is the view of the RCGP that all GPs need to consider how they achieve peer support to prevent professional isolation. For some this is a supporting practice; for others it may be a single-handed doctors group, a new practitioners group, a chambers or an educational group. Doctors who work in professional isolation miss out on many of the benefits of working in a team. They have fewer opportunities to receive or offer peer support and have fewer chances to exchange new information, which may make them feel disconnected from the profession and may make them more vulnerable to stress, exhaustion and burn-out. This may also lead to them finding it more difficult to identify areas in which they could improve their knowledge and care standards. One potential benefit of revalidation activities may be the encouragement of inter-professional linking and joint learning throughout the revalidation cycle.

2. GPs who take a break from practice in the UK

Doctors who continue to hold a licence to practise while working overseas will need to revalidate if they wish to keep their licence. They will need to connect to a UK organisation that will support them in their appraisal and revalidation. In most cases, supporting information for revalidation will need to be collected within the context of the NHS or a UK designated body, such as the defence medical services. However, it is recognised that some doctors have roles that will require them to work overseas for some periods in the revalidation cycle. We would advise that such doctors discuss their revalidation with their responsible officer or appraiser.'

So if you are in one of the unusual or isolated groups of doctors, the demands of revalidation may help bring you into more contact with your colleagues. There may actually be a positive benefit to you from revalidation. What seems like an ordeal may actually help you to become stronger professionally and richer in relationships. Sessional doctors banding together into chambers is a good move that will support many of them in their management and educational development. (Having heard this model well described by an enthusiastic 'head of chambers', I came away thinking it might be pioneering a way of working for all GPs in the future, allowing us to define our work more freely and move between roles more fluidly.)

The first thing to do is to look at the GMC's evidence requirements and see which you can achieve easily and which are a bit harder or need some lateral thinking. CPD can be achieved in many different ways and as long as it can be shown to meet a professional educational need, it counts as CPD.

The quality improvement criterion can be met through many activities – even a detailed reflective case discussion or case series discussion could be enough.

We all encounter significant events in our work; we just need to make the time to discuss them with relevant colleagues and to learn something from them.

We all have many more colleagues than we realise so obtaining MSF should be reasonably straightforward. Most sessional doctors work in a few practices only and this should enable them to become known in an area, in both primary and secondary care. Very few locums are entirely peripatetic. You may be surprised to discover how many people have observed something about your clinical practice over time.

We nearly all do surgeries and see large numbers of patients. We can all get feedback from them. We all get some complaints, and can eventually learn something from them.

With a bit of effort and ingenuity, nearly all doctors should be able to get a decent portfolio of revalidation evidence gathered together. If you are really struggling to achieve this, speak with your appraiser and RO and see what alternatives they can suggest or accept. But for most sessional GPs, the problems will be sortable.

Ultimately all doctors have to find a way to get through the requirements of revalidation. There is some local discretion for ROs and appraisers in recognising equivalence of portfolios, but the basic headings still need to be covered.

Further reading

• RCGP guide to revalidation: www.rcgp.org.uk/revalidation-and-cpd/~/media/Files/Revalidation-and-CPD/Guide%20to%20Revalidation%20v70.ashx (accessed 10 January 2013).

Reflections and background: the reasons behind revalidation

Chapter 18

Why is reflective learning so highly valued?

'Study without reflection is a waste of time. Reflection without study is dangerous.' (Confucius)

Throughout this book and in many other contexts, you will often hear the refrain about reflective learning.[1] The concept of reflection permeates all theories of adult learning and developing. Because the concept is so widely used, it risks becoming a cliché and reflection a camouflage for lazy thinking and self-justification rather than being used for learning or development.

So in this chapter I want to present the evidence and argument in favour of reflection in and on action, and hopefully show you why it is a much better way of thinking than its alternative. If you accept the need for reflective learning for yourself and your career then the concept will help you accept and use the appraisal system readily in your development.

If you think that all the talk and ideas behind reflection in action are not fully established and are in some way a waste of time and not how you learn things, then you will find processes based on reflection, such as appraisal, very difficult to accept. So this is a crucial background chapter, which I hope will provide you with reassurance that there is a developed rationale behind appraisal and revalidation, and they are not simply an annoying series of disparate tasks to complete.

My colleague Dr Ramesh Mehay, Training Programme Director of Bradford Vocational Training Scheme, has helped me with drafting this chapter, which incorporates some of the useful information he has written for the Bradford VTS website and from Chapter 28 of *The Essential Handbook for GP Training and Education* which he edited.[2]

Why do we talk so much about reflection?

I asked various colleagues this question and I got this useful brief answer from Dr Jim Lee, RO at NHS Kirklees.

'Knowledge is valuable but it only becomes truly useful when it is applied to our everyday practice. It is only when we stand back and ask ourselves "Why did I act in a certain way?, Why did I make a certain decision?, How could I have used knowledge in a better way?, What would I need to make better decisions in future?" that we start to develop our practice and ourselves meaningfully. Without this reflection the accumulation of knowledge is trophy hunting. Because effective learning won't happen unless you reflect.'

I am starting the argument in this chapter by looking at the perils that a lack of reflection brings and will then show how it can be adopted positively for your good and that of your patients.

The perils of the unreflective practitioner

I am going to go back several years and use an old-style consultant (like my dad) as an example here.

My dad did his medical training during World War II in Edinburgh and Dundee. He worked hard firstly in the army and then at Sunderland Eye Hospital and Liverpool Eye Hospital. He moved to Halifax as consultant ophthalmologist in 1967 and retired in 1990. He died in 1999 age 73.

His career was in many ways a very good one. He was likeable and liked. He inspired loyalty amongst his staff, many of whom remain family friends. He was competent; indeed, like many ophthalmologists, he was a proud, sometimes prickly, perfectionist. He was meticulous in his surgery.

As with most eye surgeons in those days, he had a long waiting list and would allow patients with cataracts to remain on his books as the cataracts 'ripened'. He had a small private practice and sent the bills out just before my school fees were due.

He was in short a very normal and decent consultant of his time, better than some, worse than others.

But when I look back further into my dad's career, I am struck by how much he had to push himself to remain good at his work. And how much it relied on his internal drives, rather than being a natural outcome of the system he worked within.

He became a consultant and after that it was assumed that he was the answer, not the question. He had done his training. It had been a tough and competitive process, that ensured the weaker ones fell by the wayside. It was a process of surviving exhaustion, developing resilience, putting up with bosses of various quality and toughness, and rather as an afterthought, some ability at your work.

He did not have an entirely enjoyable career. He was proud of his work. He worked to very high internal standards. He drove himself on. He saw many, many cases and so built up vast clinical experience. He highly valued two attributes in himself and a colleague, namely speed and accuracy.

He had no systematic review of what he was doing. He had no overview of his work and whether it was well directed or not. He had a job as a consultant ophthalmologist and he (and everyone else) knew what one of those was and what they did, and it was his duty just to do it. It kept him very busy.

He could describe his work and analyse it a little. He had no real reflection about what his work was and why it mattered; surely it was just too obvious for anyone to see that cataracts needed treating. Otherwise people would go blind. And if there were more cataracts to treat then he needed more resources to do the work. And he could only do as much as he could, and if the NHS didn't give him the means, they'd just have to put up with the inevitable waiting list. He had no sense that he could change anything much about this larger context around his work. Just a sense that he had to battle continuously against 'the collective ranks of they'. He was like many of his generation – somewhat *contra mundum* and with an internal personal inchoate scream, hidden from themselves and others under the cloak of duty. The stoicism of 'mustn't grumble' and 'that's how it is in these parts' actually has for many years reduced the NHS's internal energies towards improvement at direct patient service (as opposed to research) level.

So he ploughed on through longer and longer clinics, as many operations as he could manage, and it was clear that his duty was to keep going.

The constant treadmill of work took a toll on his health and he was ill during his fifties. His health just held out till his retirement at 65. His first advice to me when I graduated in 1989 was to buy some added years on my pension so I did not need to go on as long as he had had to.

Throughout his career, his postgraduate education was largely talking to colleagues, the hospital's Thursday lunchtime postgraduate meetings (sometimes for content, and sometimes to suss out which colleague he would go and see if he had a problem) and the North of England Ophthalmological Society meetings when he had the chance. As he got older, he was always struck by how interested registrars became when they realised he might be retiring soon and a consultant vacancy would arise.

As far as I can tell, his learning was mainly of new knowledge – new treatments, new techniques – rather than any thought about how the system, e.g his clinic scheduling, could be better arranged. He had meetings with managers about such things but they just didn't understand what was going on. The thought that it might be his duty to explain didn't seem to cross his mind. Even if he had explained he had little hope that he would have been understood.

Likewise, the idea that he could help improve referrals by teaching the local GPs some ophthalmology was foreign to him. 'They've been to medical school,' he said. The idea that most medical schools only have time to provide a brief smattering of ophthalmology teaching, and that some top-up of this for doctors in post and for whom medical school might be a receding memory, might be useful ... well, I'm not sure if he'd have liked to do it or not, but his fear of public speaking was high – he didn't have time, he didn't know what to say ..., etc.

He did not have the time or space in his work for really thinking about what he was doing, who he was working with, what skills each had and how to run the overall department well. I am not sure he would have even recognised the concepts in that sentence. As far as he was concerned, if good people came together, everything would work well. Problems were caused by laziness, incompetence or other character flaws in others. His job was to keep his own standards high and not to be bothered about the others. Registrars needed good examples, lots of cases to see and admonishment when wrong.

I think my dad was a fairly typical consultant of his age. He had a job to do and anything that took time away from that was a distraction from the real job of seeing and treating patients. When I did get him into decent discussion, he was naturally descriptive and analytical, and rarely got into deep evaluation, reflection or explanation. Everything was very factual. (Given that I am somewhat teleological and like to find out what is behind every fact I meet, this led to some friction but which father does not misunderstand his growing son?)

In short, my dad did his job, with rather little reflection about his job. I think his career failed to adapt as a result and by the end he was just about coping, but I suspect a detailed analysis could have shown some frayed edges to his work and some feeling of disappointment and of not being fully appreciated or valued. He was probably to some extent burnt out by his experiences of the NHS. He was relieved to get to his retirement, and a bit unsure what to do with it.

I use my dad's experience here to show the sort of working culture the NHS has come from. Blake Morrison's description of his GP father,[3] who would have been of a similar vintage to mine, rang many bells of recognition for me. I suspect many other old-style consultants and GPs showed very similar character traits to my dad, and that he was reasonably typical of the NHS at the time he worked within it. There is still some residue of his attitude to his work in many current doctors. It can be summed up as 'task, don't ask'. This unreflective focus on the task in hand has precluded us from asking what the task really is.

The previous culture of the NHS has been somewhat unreflective and this has led to people gritting their teeth, getting by on inner resilience and then being happy to be released into retirement. As my mother (also a doctor) commented, 'It's amazing. The people who have just retired suddenly look ten years younger'.

The new ideas about reflective practice and ongoing learning are to some extent foreign to the NHS and its workers, and have been grafted into it in addition to its many other tasks (which have not been reduced to accommodate it). This means that crucial ideas such as those summarised in Charles Vincent's book *Patient Safety*[4] are often only partially known, less understood and diminished to extra tasks, rather than considered as a basic part of the medical corpus of knowledge and praxis. Some safety-critical specialties such as anaesthetics have adopted them more readily but the significant event in the NHS as a whole is how little attention is actually paid to significant events. The North Staffordshire Enquiry is likely to make this very apparent when its report appears in 2013.

The revalidation process is forcing us to become reflective, which I think is an improvement. For many in the NHS, the reflection is

'Help, I'm so busy' and they struggle to see how they have time for reflection as well as getting the patients seen on time in the clinic. 'It's all very well for the academics in their ivory towers to invent this stuff, but when are we supposed to have the time to do it?' Actually, I would argue that if you are that busy, it is more important than ever to stop and ask yourself why you are so busy, and about how you could channel and direct the demand on you better.

Remember that you are a resourceful professional, and you probably already have most of the resources you need to solve your problems. Reflection helps you recognise these and mobilise them to make your own and your patients' lives better.

The dangerously unreflective doctor

I have just described the basic lack of reflection seen in doctors in the past and the unreflective nature of much, maybe most, activity within the NHS as a system. The doctors of those days had gained a huge amount of clinical experience but rarely reflected on it systematically.

I need now to consider a doctor with a deep and serious lack of reflection. Such doctors can be found in various places. They tend to run into medico-legal problems or disciplinary processes. They are not unintelligent. They are often working extremely hard at their job. They may well be working too much and actually trying too hard.

Their problem comes from an inability to reflect on their work. They may think their work is high quality but not bother to get the evidence about even a part of this. They may be brilliant and struggling to put up with the idiots around them. They may have other character flaws. Their basic problem will come down to an inability to handle feedback, to accept input from others or to consider that anyone apart from themselves has a valid view of a problem. Such a doctor may come across as very proud or as arrogant. Actually they are often rather fragile and very afraid of failure. The bravado is a front, rather than a reality. They demonstrate the extreme of a doctor's drive towards perfection and may want to be the finished article rather than a work in progress.

They will manage to function until a problem arises, such as a complaint. The difficulty comes when they cannot handle the negative feedback and act to deny or diminish it, rather than to deal with it.

At this stage, rather than thinking reflectively, and asking 'What happened here? What did I do to contribute to this? Is there something to learn here?', they will block reflection and learning, and show a lack of insight into the problem they are faced with. They will not grasp its nature or its potential complications. Sadly, they will then deal with it inadequately and their medical directors or medical defence advisers will be shaking their heads and saying, 'They just do not get it. I'm trying to help them and they ignore my advice'.

Just as patients are free to ignore our best advice, so too are unreflective doctors able to avoid confronting their flaws ... for a while. However, unreflective behaviour ultimately leads to lack of insight and a failure to realise when the behaviour becomes a risk to the safety of patients. And once unwillingness or inability to reflect starts raising concerns about patient safety and lack of insight, then performance concerns have arisen and have to be dealt with.

Lack of reflection is a danger sign to those concerned with professional performance that there may be a significant problem which needs investigating. One of my reasons for writing this book is to help colleagues avoid running aground on this treacherous shoreline.

The positive benefits of reflection

Up to now I have described the perils of an unreflective way of practising medicine. I now want to move away from that and show positively the benefits of a more reflective style of practice, both for you personally and in terms of patient outcomes. And as Hart et al. point out,[2] many doctors have heard of reflection but few have been taught how to do it well.

The classic description of reflection is derived from the work of Donald Schön.[1] He described the idea that we both reflect *on* action (after the event) and reflect whilst we are *in* action (thinking on our feet). There is a lovely section near the beginning of his book where he describes the crisis he perceives in professional knowledge:

'In the varied topography of professional practice, there is a high, hard ground overlooking a swamp. On the high ground, manageable problems lend themselves to solution through the application of research-based theory and technique. In the swampy lowland, messy, confusing problems defy technical solutions. The irony of this situation is that the problems of the high ground tend to be relatively unimportant to individuals or society at large, however great their technical interest may be, while in the swamp lie the problems of greatest human concern. The practitioner must choose. Shall he remain on the high ground where he can solve relatively unimportant problems according to prevailing standards of rigor, or shall he descend to the swamp of important problems and non-rigorous enquiry?'

He asserts that the only way to manage the 'indeterminate zones of practice' is through the ability to think on your feet, and apply previous experience to new situations. But for Schön, it wasn't just about creating knowledge. Professionals also have to use their knowledge, and look back critically on their actions.

Most doctors will recognise the split behind the clear view from the high ground and the messy reality of day-by-day practice. Reflection is one practical way of lifting ourselves out of our current swamp, and getting some of the clearer view from the uplands to help us in our next journey through the swamp. Reflection and learning are a way of integrating our practice with theory and other knowledge, and getting a better overall understanding of what we do and why we do it. The old ways of excessive experience and too little reflection will now seem unattractive but too much reflection on too little experience will also be unsatisfactory. Neither the omphaloscope nor the retrospectoscope is a satisfactory instrument of discovery.

Your appraisal interview is one day in the year when you can emerge from the swamp and see how things look from the sunlit uplands, at least for a brief time. The real work of medicine is done in the swamp, and our unique selling point as doctors is the combination of knowledge, skill, tenacity and compassion that enables us to help our patients navigate the messiness of day-by-day medicine well and safely. In your appraisal interview, you can for a while reflect on how well you help your patients to do this. Every so often, it is worth reminding ourselves how much medicine does actually go right, despite the many ways in which it could go wrong. Reflection can bring light to bear on both what goes well and what goes less well, and can help us define problems, both in terms of what they are and also against what background you are noticing them.

Kemmis[5] states that reflection is more than a process that focuses 'on the head'. It is a positive active process that reviews, analyses and evaluates experiences, draws on theoretical concepts or previous learning and so provides an action plan for future experiences. Johns[6] adds that reflection is a personal process that enables the practitioner to assess understand and learn through their experiences. This results in some change in their perspective of a situation or creates new learning for the individual.

Ultimately the outcome of reflection is learning. Reflection widens our perspective on a problem (breadth). It helps us develop strategies for dealing with it (developing skills). It helps us acquire new insights into our behaviour (attitudes change). In short, a doctor who is demonstrating some form of reflective practice is demonstrating learning, and a capacity to self-improve. A doctor who is not doing this sort of activity is falling behind his or her peers.

Some doctors do question the value of reflection, or say they do it but only very quickly, and do not write it down. Hart *et al.*[2] review these objections well, as does Clark[7] in a piece provocatively titled 'Let's reflect: what is the point?'. Well, the point is learning, and good doctors are good learners. Good learners also tend to be good teachers.

The revalidation system insists on us providing some basic evidence of reflection, and I hope from what I have described so far about why unreflective practice is bad for us, and how reflection is a positive way of learning that you can see why reflection is so highly valued.

Key qualities and skills required for proper reflection

Commitment to self-enquiry and readiness to change practice are important if the individual is to get the most out of the process. The qualities needed include:

- open-mindedness
- commitment to self-enquiry
- motivation
- readiness to change practice.

The skills needed include[7]:

- *information* – describing what happened or what was observed in enough but not too much detail
- *self-awareness* – being open and honest about performance but also writing about own feelings and/or those of others
- *critical thinking* – analysing the bigger and smaller pictures, problem solving, describing own thought processes

- *evaluation* – pooling the above three things (synthesis) and describing what needs to be learned, why and how.

Levels or depths of reflection – ISCE levels

Various levels of reflection have been described.[2,8] The purely descriptive elements are a starting point but not enough on their own. Four levels of reflection have been described using the acronym ISCE:

- Information provided

- Self-awareness

- Critical analysis

- Evidence for learning.

In training and in appraisals, we are looking for evidence of the deeper levels of reflection. Mere cataloguing and description is not enough – it is just the start. It is from the reflection on what has gone well and what has gone not so well that the learning and insight emerge.

How do we learn to reflect more deeply?

The levels above give some good hints about what is involved in proper reflection. Sadly, in revalidation, it is possible to be unreflectively reflective – to make it look as if you are reflecting, when in fact all you are doing is getting through your appraisal.

Some doctors are not naturally given to reflection and find reflection in action rather a trial.[2,7] Some doctors are naturally reflective but they do it so quickly that they think, 'I'm not into this reflective learning. I just spot the gap in knowledge and fill it immediately'.

Kolb's experiential learning cycle is a useful model for some.[9] Different doctors prefer different parts of this cycle but in appraisal and revalidation, you are encouraged to visit all the parts of the cycle. The cycle describes four key parts, namely experiencing, reflecting, conceptualising and experimenting.

- *Concrete experience* is about something that has happened to you or that you have done.

- *Reflection* is concerned with reviewing the event or experience and exploring what you did and how you and others felt about it.

- *Abstract conceptualisation* is all about developing an understanding of what happened by seeking more information or bringing in theoretical concepts or previous learning to form new ideas about ways of doing things in the future.

- *Active experimentation* is about trying these newly formed ideas.

Broadly this corresponds to:

- What happened?

- What do I think and/or feel about this?

- What more general concepts do I bring to this reflection? What is this event an example of?

- What will I do differently next time? What happens when I try my new strategy out?

When reflecting-on-action, the first step in the process is the description of the incident. The key thing in appraisal is to check that the description of the event is accurate, and then to move beyond it. In philosophical terms, epistemology comes before hermaneutics. Or more simply, the first questions are epistemic – 'How do I know that I know this?' and 'How might I have got this wrong?'.[10,11] Having checked the description, then the second question is hermaneutic – 'How do I know what this means?'. In a science context, it is the difference between the methods and results section of a paper, and the ensuing discussion.

The better we can do reflection, the more we can move from mere description to deeper understanding of ourselves and our work. And ultimately deepening our understanding of our work is the worthwhile outcome of appraisal processes. All the supporting information we bring to the process is only useful if there is some reflective learning process applied to it. Without it, the information is just data, lacking context, explanation or meaning.

Do you really want to make your appraisal or your career a meaningless process? A merely technical way of passing the time and earning an income? I do not think that many doctors would want that, and so I propose that we should celebrate reflection-in-action, and use the process well for our own learning and our own improvement, and to help towards developing better service for patients.

Plato said that the unexamined life is not worth living. Perhaps for us as doctors, the unexamined profession is not worth maintaining. Perhaps appraisal should be seen as our chance to examine our life and work in a protected setting.

References

1   Schön D. *The Reflective Practitioner.* London: Kogan Page; 1984.
2   Hart J, Waters M, Rughani A, Mehay R. Reflection and evaluation. In: *The Essential Handbook for GP Training and Education.* London: Radcliffe Publishing; 2012.
3   Morrison B. *And When Did You Last See Your Father?* London: Penguin; 2007.
4   Vincent C. *Patient Safety.* Oxford: Blackwell; 2010.
5   Kemmis S. Action research and the politics of reflection. In: Boud D, Keogh R, Walker D, editors. *Turning Learning into Experience.* London: Kogan Page; 1985.
6   Johns C. The value of reflective learning for nursing. *J Clin Nursing.* 1995; **4**: 23–60.
7   Clark J. Let's reflect: what is the point? *Br J Gen Pract.* 2011; **61**: 747.
8   Richardson G, Maltby H. Reflection on practice: enhancing student learning. *J Adv Nursing.* 1995; **22**: 235–42.
9   Kolb A, Kolb DA. *Experiential Learning. Experience as a source of learning and development.* New Jersey: Prentice-Hall; 1984.
10 Schultz K. *Being Wrong: adventures in the margin of error.* London: Portobello Books; 2010.
11 Sutherland S. *Irrationality: the enemy within.* London: Penguin; 1992.

Chapter 19

Some thoughts on feedback

This chapter is a reflective essay on feedback, and its good and bad points. It is for debate and consideration. As far as revalidation goes, we all will be giving and receiving feedback no matter how well or badly it is done. (If you have paid attention to the earlier chapters, it will hopefully be done well.)

This chapter takes the consideration of feedback to a deeper level, beyond the merely practical task of getting through revalidation. Its key point is that the recipient of feedback needs to understand the quality and validity or weakness of the feedback they are receiving. Knowing how to receive feedback, and which bits to incorporate into ourselves and which bits to discard, is an unrecognised art.

For ease of understanding, I use 'I' and 'you' as the two people involved in the conversation. I am sure you can transpose the pronouns appropriately to your own context.

On giving and receiving feedback

If feedback is truly the breakfast of champions, how come I sometimes get indigestion when I receive it?

We live in a feedback age and revalidation is all about feedback and reflection. We are enjoined by the GMC and others to be ever more accountable, to achieve goals and targets, and generally both to be more productive and to demonstrate that we are being more productive. Power has christened it 'the audit society'.[1] It is a strange world in which it is at least as, and probably more, important to represent your activity well as to actually just get on and do it well.[2] It can appear as if we all now need our personal version of Alistair Campbell, to present a good facade and to hide any rotting carcasses.

93

Someone is always watching you and will be offering you 'feedback'. Enoch Powell used to comment that all political lives would end in failure and I think with the increasing scrutiny, and the shifting sands of official thinking, most professional lives will end in failure.

At some level all this feedback is good, as it should encourage us to be better people both at being and doing. The days of the isolated single-handed doctor or the village teacher ploughing their own furrows of idiosyncrasy or idiocy for many years before retiring do not seem great days to go back to. As Swensen *et al.* commented in the *New England Journal of Medicine*, we are moving from the days of 'cottage industry' to the days of postindustrial care.[3]

As Mary Midgley describes, we are primarily social beings, not individuals, and we only learn in contact with others.[4] Even a sage meditating alone on a mountain can only justify this aloneness by coming down and telling us what he has discovered later.

And yet I still have very mixed feelings about feedback, and the people who I allow to give me feedback. I am not sure how useful it is, either to me or my organisation. Nor am I always entirely clear to what purpose the feedback is being given. I am not always sure I really want feedback, and this may be a flaw in me rather than you.

I want to explore in this essay why I have some problems and reservations around feedback. As the old school grace puts it, 'For what we are about to receive, may the Lord make us truly thankful' and sadly, I am sometimes about as grateful for feedback as a five year old with a plate of sprouts and broccoli.

I will be as honest as possible here about what is my personal baggage, but as many psychologists put it, 'that which is most personal is also the most general'. The closer I can get to my core, the closer I also come to yours. I may succeed in showing in this essay what the basis for this claim is. Also when I comment on others, I am aware that what I say about others may say as much about me as it does about them. If I point out the splinter in your eye, whilst missing the plank in my own, please be gentle correcting me, as you may be doing just the same in reverse. As the Americans put it, 'Oh Lord, please make my words as sweet as honey, as tomorrow I may need to eat them'.

The French phenomenological philosopher Maurice Merleau-Ponty points out that no perception comes to us without having a meaning already assigned to it.[5] We are conditioned, whether by nature or by nurture, to sort for difference and to pay most attention to threats and difficulties, and because of this we rarely stop to celebrate what is good, stable and reliable in the overall picture. Pendleton *et al.*'s helpful rules about feedback – and about paying attention to the good points first – consciously correct for this tendency but sadly these are not universally honoured.[6]

The inner and outer aspects of life

The core of feedback is that your perceptions and mine have to mix and merge to some extent. There is a dynamic equilibrium between our internal and external axes of thought and evaluation and this equilibrium can easily be unbalanced by either side.

There are four key corners that set the field for this balance. From my side, there is a continuum between me validating myself and me invalidating myself. From your side, there is a continuum between you validating me and you invalidating me. There is a balance, an Aristotelian golden mean to be struck to avoid getting stuck at any extreme.

We need to look along the axes first of all to see the problems there.

Me invalidating me

This is the classic terrain of psychotherapy. The classic themes of low self-esteem, low personal confidence, victim states, 'poor little me', dominate here. My thought processes here are self-sabotaging, full of unjustified fears, and also tending to give servile, fawning and excessive value to what others say about me. Dylan Thomas captures the dynamics of this state beautifully in *Under Milk Wood*.[7,8] The whole play is dominated by the dreadful fear about 'What'll the neighbours think/say …?' and the even worse fear of finding out exactly what they are saying.

Doctors tend to be overdriven perfectionists and to a large extent, many of us are driven by a powerful fear of failure and of letting others down. We may appear confident but often our confidence is overplayed, and can come over as arrogance when actually what is going on is a fear of appearing incompetent or ridiculous. There is a lot of 'keeping up appearances' going on in medicine, and it can result in some unpleasant and unco-operative behaviours.

We may, like other humans, be incapable of assimilating and accepting too much reality at once, and feedback brings the risk of this happening rather quickly. We may simultaneously need the feedback from others to grow, and recoil in fear from accepting it.

There is a fair amount of psychopathology to our healing enterprise and we would do well to acknowledge its existence.[9-12] The price of not doing so is too high, personally for doctors, and risky for our patients. (Appendix 1 gives some helpful advice about this.)

Me validating me

Justified confidence and accurate self-knowledge are valuable gifts and need to be used well, and protected from unjustified criticism.

The overbalance of this is excessive confidence in myself, tending towards arrogance and pig-headedness. I might think all I am doing is right, and you might be desperately trying to warn me of an impending disaster, but I will dismiss your opinions with 'What do you know anyway?'. Behaviour at this end of the scale is immediately unattractive and potentially dangerous, and unless I am right all the way through, you may take great delight to see my eventual fall.

In our colleague and patient feedback for revalidation, we are asked to rate ourselves and then compare our ratings against those who give us feedback. Most doctors tend to mark themselves down and blush modestly when their friends and colleagues rate them more highly than they do themselves. There is a mixture of politeness and false modesty at work here.

As appraisers and ROs, we get more worried if we see poor doctors overestimating their skill and competence, and maintaining this forcefully even in the face of negative feedback. Phrases like 'lack of insight' and 'inability to empathise with others' start to emerge.

You validating me

The experience of encouragement, and shared experience, can be very good feedback. It shows shared perspectives and realisations and that my perspective is not merely personal or parochial. It is hopefully an example of great minds thinking alike rather than fools seldom differing.

The flip side of this is when you give me fulsome praise for something minor and not really deserving of the praise. If you give me too much praise, and I am vain enough to accept it, we are both fools together. The danger here is that when I realise that you were giving me excessive praise, and the final outcome is not as good as you led me to expect, I will turn on you and blame you for my failings.

The recipient of feedback needs to be able to evaluate the quality of the feedback, possibly to a higher degree than the person giving it needs to know how to give it. We underestimate our need to learn about how best to prepare ourselves to receive feedback, both from an improvement and a self-protection viewpoint.

You invalidating me

This need for protection is even greater if your feedback to me is negative. That is, that I am either doing something wrong or need to alter my behaviour in some way. You may be absolutely right to give me such feedback but I may react by shooting the messenger. Justified criticism is very good feedback and although uncomfortable to receive, is valuable. Only a true friend can deliver this form of feedback well, and their efforts are likely to be appreciated only later, rather than immediately.

I think I go through a grief reaction when I receive negative feedback, and follow all the Kübler-Ross stages of[13]:

- *anger* – how dare you say that about this? Or about me myself?

- *grief* – how could you say that about this?

- *bargaining* – surely it's not as bad as all that?

- *denial* – I don't see any problem with this

- *acceptance* – OK so this isn't great, but I'll see what I can do to improve it.

I have a bad habit of immediately perceiving negative feedback as being personal, permanent and pervasive and it sometimes takes me a while to get around to acceptance. I'll bet many of my readers are like that too, and take a while to get around to reframing the problem as a learning opportunity.

The overbalance of justified criticism is the 'hatchet job' – feedback that is personal, *ad hominem*, an attack on my beliefs and values, often coming from a different map of reality, with no attempt at explanation. Often such ferocious attacks come from an unrecognised fear in the person giving feedback, and usually say more about them than whatever the feedback is supposedly about. Classic examples in medicine are:

- when I want your opinion I'll give it to you

- you'll go far with that attitude

- you'll never work in this town again

- a modest man with much to be modest about

- I'd comment on his work – if he'd ever done any

- he carried out his duties entirely to his satisfaction

- let me tell you!

We need to be able to spot this type of feedback and not take it personally. This involves some degree of disassociation and a mental move to higher ground from where it can be viewed at a distance and seen for what it is, and not be associated with or incorporated into ourselves. Such feedback is toxic, and we need a way to decontaminate it. Whether this should be achieved by the recipient of the feedback or be moderated by another is not yet clear. The possibility of such feedback is why there are fears around the implementation of colleague and patient feedback in the revalidation process.

Why I tend to take feedback personally

The classic advice on feedback is to keep it at the level of observable behaviour and not to address it to the person directly. I think this is good advice but even if it is followed scrupulously, I may still take it personally. The reason for this is that my behaviour is the result of my thoughts and beliefs. So if there is criticism of my behaviour, there is also by inference (me bringing into myself) criticism of the thoughts and beliefs behind the behaviour.

Simply saying 'please don't take this personally' guarantees that it will be, just as you were not thinking about a pink giraffe but you are now that I have told you not to think of a pink giraffe.

To some extent I will take all feedback personally. I don't know to what extent my experience is typical of others.

Why I used to struggle to accept compliments

The flip side of being wary about receiving feedback is the difficulty I used to have about accepting compliments. My wife picked this up in me and since her intervention, if someone gives me a compliment, I simply accept it with thanks. A sincerely meant compliment is great feedback and should be accepted at face value.

Purposes of feedback

As far as I can tell, there has to be a purpose to giving feedback. Feedback involves you sharing your take on reality with me and for you to do that is itself a sign that I matter to you. Thank you for that. The only thing worse than feedback is no feedback at all!

To my mind, there are some key questions that arise from the four quadrants described above.

Me validating me

How far can I go in believing that I am right?

How justified is my confidence?

Me invalidating me

Can I even get started if I won't believe in me?

And why should I get started anyway?

And if I won't believe in myself, why should you?

You validating me

How far, or how much further, can I go if you are giving me positive feedback?

You invalidating me

How can I go on in the face of external criticism?

Have I missed something?

Have you not spotted something?

Do I need to consider whether I am mistaken?

On the quality of feedback itself

The quality of feedback is an issue in its own right. It is independent of the subject or object of the feedback itself. If we consider feedback on a given action, the action itself may be good or bad and the feedback about the action might be good or bad.

- Good feedback about a good action takes the form of deserved praise.

- Bad feedback about a good action could be either unjustified condemnation or false praise.

- Good feedback about a bad action takes the form of justified, well-judged criticism.

- Bad feedback about a bad action is usually excessive judgement, *ad hominem*, or an unnecessary retaliation. Or even more deadly, false praise.

As always, the goal is the Aristotelian aim of achieving the right action for the right reason at the right time and in the right place.

In feedback scenarios, you can end up getting the right feedback despite the wrong reasons or the wrong motives in either yourself or others. You could also end up receiving the wrong feedback despite the best motives and reasons in either yourself or others.

In short, receiving the right message about yourself at the right time and in the right way is an art form in itself. I know I have not mastered this yet for myself or for others. I doubt that others have mastered it fully either. Who amongst us lives free of the good or bad opinions of others?[8] Whom do we trust to give us good feedback, and whom do we distrust with feedback? It is worth asking yourself who you will allow to speak into your life, and why you will accept their input but not someone else's? Suggested criteria for allowing others to speak into your life include respect for their knowledge, abilities or character, respect for their achievements (especially if you want to emulate them) or respect for their outcomes. Of course, in revalidation, we have to accept feedback from the many and varied colleagues around us, rather than from our intellectual and professional heroes. But in terms of your own development (as opposed to the minor task of getting through revalidation), it is well worth thinking about who you will allow to speak to you and influence you. And about who you will keep away from your development.

To what extent should this be the responsibility of the feedback giver to arrange? Or is it the responsibility of the feedback recipient to prepare for receiving the feedback?

What feedback is really all about

Feedback is both a vital and a challenging problem and opportunity for us all. It is vital and challenging both to the giver and the recipient. It occurs at the boundary between our private and public selves, which is one of the key balance points in all our lives.

As humans, we are a part of the reality that we experience. We are both embodied and 'enminded' and we have at least three parts to our maps of reality in play at any one time.[5,13] These are:

- our map of external reality (how the world happens for and to us, our sense of the world)

- our map of our internal reality (our sense of ourselves)

- our external presentation (our presentation of ourselves to the world, how we happen to the world).

All these maps are approximations and we have to generalise, delete and distort reality as the whole of it at once would simply overwhelm us. And we cannot know the world as it is in itself, we can only know it as it seems to us.[14] Feedback is set at the point where our internal and external maps of reality meet. Feedback may validate or invalidate our experiences, perspectives and beliefs. How do I know that this is how it is for me? For you? For everybody else?

Your feedback to me may open up or close down my map of reality. It may recover some of my deletions, generalisations and distortions and so enrich my map. Or it may simply allow you to pass some of your generalisations, deletions and distortions onto me ('let me tell you, my boy!'). The mote in my perception may actually be a plank in yours ('and let me tell you just how much more you've missed yourself, dear').

You give feedback to me from your maps of reality to my maps of reality. What you spot in me you have already noticed for yourself. You may very well be a pot calling my kettle black, and you'll probably be right to do so ... but have you noticed your own blackness? The way in which you give me feedback will of itself give me a very clear idea about you and how you relate to the world.

Feedback is such a finely balanced and two-way process that both giver and receiver are in fact giving and receiving from each other, moment by moment throughout the whole game. If you are not learning as you give feedback, you are not giving feedback, you are simply dictating or instructing.

Feedback done well is two people coming to understand themselves and their world better. It brings our internal and external realities into sharp focus. It allows us to align our inner and outer takes on reality and so to re-anchor ourselves in reality. It prevents us going off on flights of fancy and chasing grand abstractions that will never be grounded in anyone else's reality. The ability to receive and assimilate feedback is actually a sign of sanity and the inability to handle feedback is a sign of madness.

I want to conclude with this quote from the *Gospel of Thomas* that for me sums up feedback beautifully.

'When you make the two one,
when you make the inner as the outer,
and the outer as the inner ...
Then you shall enter the Kingdom.'

References

1   Power M. *The Audit Society. Rituals of verification*. Oxford: OUP; 1999.
2   Kenny A, Davies P. *Probophilia – a disease of our time*. 2010. www.civitas.org.uk/nhs/download/probophilia.pdf
3   Swensen SJ, Meyer GS, Nelson EC, *et al*. Cottage industry to postindustrial care – the revolution in healthcare delivery. *N Engl J Med*. 2010; **362**: e12.
4   Midgley M. *The Myths We Live By*. London: Routledge: 2004.
5   Merleau-Ponty M. The perceptual faith and reflection. In: *The Visible and The Invisible*. Evanston, IL: Northwestern University Press; 1968. pp. 28–49.
6   Pendleton D, Schofield T, Tate P, Havelock P. *The New Consultation: developing doctor–patient communication*. 2nd ed. Oxford: OUP; 2003.
7   Thomas D. *Under Milk Wood*. London: BBC; 1953.
8   Davies P. Answering the neighbours. *Caduceus*. 2002; **57**: 34–5.
9   Ghodse H, Mann S, Johnson P, editors. *Doctors and their Health*. Sutton, Surrey: Reed Business Information; 2000.
10 Siebert A. *The Resiliency Advantage: master change, thrive under pressure, and bounce back from setbacks*. San Francisco, CA: Berrett-Koehler; 2005.
11 Bennet G. *The Wound and the Doctor: healing, technology and power in modern medicine*. London: Secker & Warburg; 1987.
12 Rowe L, Kidd M. *First Do No Harm: being a resilient doctor in the 21st century*. Maidenhead: McGraw-Hill Medical; 2009.
13 Kübler-Ross E. *On Death and Dying*. London: Routledge: 1969.
14 Davies P. The radical accuracy of the subjective viewpoint. *Br J Gen Pract*. 2007; 57: 848–9.

Chapter 20

How can revalidation benefit me?

Many doctors are somewhat cynical about revalidation. They see it as an imposition on the profession and 'just another flipping thing' on the ever-growing 'to do' list. Some see it is as unfair, or biased, or as a witch hunt aiming to drive certain groups of doctors out of the profession. Some are using it as an excuse to bring forward their retirement. May I suggest a different and much more positive narrative?

Revalidation means 'to make strong again'. Revalidation will make us strong again, both individually and as part of our collective profession.

The fact that we willingly undergo this process is to our personal and professional credit. It will be a clear sign to the public that their doctor cares about their professional standards and their need to continually be improving them. This will make it very difficult for any politician, or other outside observer, to accuse the profession of being 'doctor centred' or simply a 'vested producer interest'. Revalidation will demonstrate a depth of concern about our processes and standards that other observers will struggle to match. It can help us raise the credibility of our profession, which after the attacks it suffered in the late 1990s and early 2000s does need raising again.[1]

Being a valued member of a very valuable profession must be good for our personal and collective morale. For us as individual doctors, the value of the process is not in the revalidation decision, it is in the processes of thought and reflection that lead up to that decision. As in most activities in life, the effort you put in will be the value you get out of it. You can do the minimum and scrape through or you can pursue your postgraduate education as something worth doing both for its own sake and to improve your care to patients. Either way, the standard is sufficiently challenging to be useful but not so high as to make revalidation hard.

We will learn more as we go through revalidation, and its focus on continually finding gaps and problems and remedying them will almost inevitably lead to us becoming system leaders as well as doctors, as we will become the main agents for change and improvement within the NHS. The last 20 years or so of NHS history have seen a growth of managerialism, which to a large extent has been ranged as a force against doctors.[2,3] The NHS is now coming to realise that, like any other knowledge-based industry, it must have its main people with technical knowledge helping to set up and run the system. In a German engineering company the managers work alongside the engineers, not against them. In the future of the NHS, this needs to happen again, and the signs are that managers now realise that the NHS will not work if managers and doctors are ranged against each other. This simply gives the managers an impossible job doing something they don't understand and the doctors a miserable job as they feel unappreciated. Aneurin Bevan realised this at the start of the NHS, as shown in this quote.

> 'After all – I need not remind you of this – I am a Socialist and, being a Socialist, I believe in industrial democracy, and because I believe in industrial democracy I believe that doctors as a profession must have a greater and greater say in the management of their own services.' (Aneurin Bevan, 1945)

Perhaps it is time for us to command, through respect, a greater and greater say in the management of our own services. And maybe revalidation is a key to achieving this.

For individual doctors, owning the processes of quality improvement in their surgeries and departments will increase their sense of ownership and responsibility for their work. It gives us all a lead into clinical leadership,[4] and the perfect excuse to sort out problems where they are found. There is now official encouragement from the NHS and GMC structures for an approach which emphasises problem sorting, rather than problem ignoring or hoping someone else will do something about it.

If as doctors we rediscover the confidence to start sorting out problems in our workplaces, then we may well move from 'just working here' and 'it's a job' to a renewed sense of pride in our work. There are great possibilities here and this process actually gives us encouragement to revalidate our self-belief as doctors. Although to some extent revalidation is being imposed on us, it does contain a significant opportunity for our profession, which we can exploit to our own and our patients' benefits. Let's realise that we have an opportunity here.

References

1 Irvine D. Patients, professionalism and revalidation. *BMJ*. 2005; **330:** 1265–8.
2 Davies P, Gubb J. *Putting Patients Last*. London: Civitas; 2009.
3 Klein R. *The New Politics of the NHS*. 6th ed. London: Radcliffe Publishing; 2010.
4 Davies P, Moran L, Gandhi H. Leadership. In: *The New GP's Handbook*. London: Radcliffe Publishing; 2012.

Chapter 21

Does revalidation actually achieve its objective?

'Time will say nothing but I told you so,
Time only knows the price we have to pay:
If I could tell you I would let you know.' (Auden)

There is a quality to the consideration of revalidation that is well captured by the ambivalence of Auden's poem. We now know the structure of revalidation, and have some idea of the price we have to pay, but we do not yet know if there is any value to the process or not.

So far this book has mostly been descriptive, about processes and procedures that if followed will keep you away from trouble. If I have successfully shown you these, and you are now confident about what to do and how to do it, I will have made your own, your appraiser's and your RO's lives easier and the book will have achieved its purpose. And you will get through revalidation quickly and easily.

In this final chapter, I want to ask a more evaluative question which looks at whether revalidation will achieve its purpose.

The first thing we need to do is to remind ourselves that revalidation is meant to ensure that doctors are 'fit to practise and up to date'. Will revalidation achieve this? And following on from this, will getting doctors to this standard improve the service that patients receive?

These are apparently simple questions but getting a clear answer to them is not easy. Revalidation is not a simple exercise and it is not an obviously self-validating concept.

I could argue the negative here quite forcefully – namely that a doctor who is not taking part in the activities of quality improvement, SEA,

CPD, colleague and patient feedback, and reviewing complaints and compliments is probably a poor doctor. These processes are basic to any doctor's reflection about their practice, and a doctor who is not even meeting these minimal criteria is unlikely to be practising in a safe and reflective manner, and is unlikely to be learning from mistakes and feedback. So I can say that if these processes are not in place then it is likely the doctor is not thinking clearly or performing well, and that this may be putting their patients at risk.

But I am not sure that the positive case for revalidation is yet made. There is no randomised trial of doctors who have been through the process comparing their standards with doctors who have not undertaken this process. We can do natural observations of what happens before and after revalidation is introduced, but such observational cohorts have inbuilt biases (selection, recall, etc.) and are not fully convincing evidence that revalidation works.

At one level, revalidation is a statutory process written into the GMC's procedures and we as doctors have to lump it and get on with it. It would be nicer if we were sure the process was fully validated.

We do not have gold standard randomised control trial evidence about revalidation as a therapeutic intervention. We do not know scientifically whether doctors who have been through revalidation perform better clinically than those who have not been through such a process. Revalidation is an untrialled intervention, based on educational and regulatory theory rather than experimental confirmation. It may in time come to be seen as the educational and regulatory processes' version of mannitol, and maintenance of the colloid oncotic pressure in volume replacement. (For those of you young enough not to have heard of mannitol, it was used for many years in an attempt to restore colloid oncotic pressure in volume depletion/fluid replacement scenarios, and the physiology suggested that there was a need to balance colloid against crystalloid fluid volume replacement. Eventually, randomised controlled trials showed that mannitol added nothing to the crystalloid fluid replacement, and may even have been dangerous.)

Revalidation may work as a process by persuading some older or less competent doctors that they do not want to go through with it, so that they withdraw voluntarily from the GMC Register and retire earlier than they otherwise would have done. This may represent over-harsh self-perception by some doctors (who otherwise would have gone on to provide good service to patients – a significant loss of knowledge and experience). Alternatively, it may be insightful self-criticism and a realisation by these doctors that they are not fully up to date or accurate in their practice, and that it is time that they call it a day (thus leaving with their reputation intact and reducing the risk to patients from doctors who are not up to date or fit to practise). The days of retired doctors being dusted down and brought in to do locums for 'a few weeks in the summer holidays' are now going, and the fixed costs of medicine such as meeting revalidation criteria, medical defence and registration costs make such postretirement dabbling all but impossible. In future, we will either work as doctors or be clearly out of practice.

For some doctors over 55, particularly in primary care, the current (2012–13) combination of static or falling personal incomes, higher National Insurance and pensions contributions and then revalidation and commissioning requirements on top is making the decision to retire earlier rather than later a fairly straightforward one. Fundamentally, they are seeing their combination of satisfaction, salary and support tilting in an unfavourable direction. If this trend gathers pace, we will lose a lot of medical wisdom and capacity from the NHS, and may not be able to replace it quickly enough.

The revalidation and appraisal processes may allow medical directors and responsible officers to spot people in actual or potential trouble earlier and so bring remedial processes into play, before disciplinary and performance management concerns arise. In this way, the process may head off much regulatory and GMC trouble before it can get started. The process can help focus the system's attention onto failing doctors, before they damage either themselves or their patients. The days of doctors being good despite the system they work in should be going. We should now be moving to a system that cares about us as doctors, and helps us to become better doctors and keep away from trouble. Yes, some doctors will fall foul of regulatory processes, but it would be good to keep this number to the minimum possible. Medical directors are in a bind – they care about high standards of medical practice, and they mostly like their colleagues. They know how to launch performance investigations but they would much rather not have to go through such processes. Appraisal and revalidation may save them having to launch as many performance investigations, and may instead allow them to act to head off trouble so that their colleagues keep on practising and the patients keep on getting good service.

Medical directors would prefer to nudge you towards good performance if they possibly can. For us as individual doctors, we want our work environments to have their 'choice architecture' fashioned in such a way that it is easier for us to do the right thing properly, rather than take a risky short cut just to get the job done quickly enough.

I can think of some appraisals I have done that have headed off major partnership rifts or facilitated reflection which then allowed a doctor to make a significant move or change so that potential danger to the doctor was avoided. The days of bickering partners in a practice or consultants at loggerheads in a small department, soldiering on trying to maintain a service when the partnership or department was failing, may be going, and the appraisal process may be a means by which the need for necessary moves is identified sooner rather than later. And hopefully before either the doctor's health is impaired or harm has been done to patients. But I am not sure that anybody could show such an effect positively – it will all be anecdotes and observations, and very difficult to measure. And all such stories will have at least two sides – the dysfunctional partnership or department may well think the departing doctor is the dysfunctional element and that things will go back to 'normal' now that he or she has gone.

There are many, such as Greenhalgh and Wong,[1] who worry that revalidation risks becoming over-technical and privileging the bureaucratic and technical side of medicine over the more humane side. But we need to acknowledge that this tension between the technical and caring sides of the medical endeavour has always been present. It is embodied in the RCGP motto *Cum scientia caritas* (Knowledge with compassion). We have always needed to be able to hear a heart murmur, whether as a valve lesion or a sign of a broken heart. And we cannot hope to measure all aspects of medicine at once.

Some people doubt whether the process will work at all. Nigel Hawkes summarised the doubts well in a November 2012 *BMJ* article.[2] He sees the long development phase (since 1998) as evidence that the idea is not fully convincing to many. He thinks the costs of the process itself and the number of doctors who will need remediation or disciplinary measures are unknown and unknowable. He thinks that revalidation may be offering, or pretending to offer, something it cannot deliver. He's also unsure about whether finding the 1% of problem doctors makes it worthwhile bothering the 99% of doctors whom you are not concerned about. The answer to his doubts is something along the lines of 'do we employ more policemen to catch more criminals, or do we try to raise the standard of lawfulness amongst citizens so that more police are not needed?'. Which approach is best suited to raising standards of medical practice and protecting patients from harm is still not clear.

Revalidation is at the least an attempt to ensure that doctors are fit to practise and up to date. It will not make every doctor perfect overnight. It will not mean that all treatment is perfectly directed. What it will do is at least ensure that some basic items of ongoing development are in place, and that some form of reflection and learning is happening. As a teacher once put it about his pupils, 'At least I try to get the b******s to think'.

Maybe revalidation at least tries to get us some time and space to think. And insists that such activity is time well spent and not merely a way of missing a clinic or operating list. And that the system must act to support and encourage such educational and appraisal activity, and not see it as a soft expenditure, that can easily be cut.

Anyhow, whatever you think of it, the revalidation process is with us now and as a doctor, you need to understand it and what it is asking of you, and what you need to do about it and for it. If it works, it will strengthen you as an individual doctor and strengthen the system, as all its doctors will be fit to practise and up to date. This high quality of individual doctors is such a key component of the patient experience that this should lead to improvements in the quality of care that patients receive.

I hope it will succeed in achieving this outcome which would be good for doctors, the profession, our patients and the NHS as a whole. We will find out whether it does achieve this over the next five years or so.

References

1   Greenhalgh T, Wong G. Revalidation: a critical perspective. *Br J Gen Pract.* 2011; **61**(584): 166–8.
    http://qmro.qmul.ac.uk/jspui/handle/123456789/2239 (accessed 17 December 2012).
2   Hawkes N. Revalidation seems to add little to the current appraisal process. *BMJ.* 2012; **345**: e7375. http://dx.doi.org/10.1136/bmj.e7375 (accessed 17 December 2012).

How to stay sane and healthy as a doctor

This chapter is drawn from an earlier book, *The New GP's Handbook*.[1] It is relevant to revalidation, as it shows you why the health declaration is so important, why it is so important to make it accurately, and the risks of getting it wrong.

There are specific issues and concerns around our health as doctors which deserve to be known and considered, and hopefully mostly handled before they cause us problems and any harm to our patients. Medicine is a stressful occupation and although most of us handle this stress well, we do this at some cost to ourselves, our relationships and our health.

Revalidation is a current stress on many doctors, and I think that the information and advice in this chapter may be timely for many readers.

'Show me a sane man and I will cure him for you.' (C.G. Jung)

'The patient is the one with the disease.'[2]

Why does a doctor's health matter?

Doctors are an unusual group of patients. We know a lot but we are not very good at applying our knowledge to ourselves. We deal with patients well and mostly find it a straightforward process. It is what we are trained to do. When it comes to applying our knowledge to our own symptoms, we are rarely accurate and yet we are often reluctant to ask a colleague to run his or her well-trained medical gaze over us. It is often difficult for us as caregivers to become the receivers of care.

113

As the old saying has it, 'a doctor who treats himself has a fool for a patient'.

In some ways doctors can be seen as a group whose health needs are poorly catered for. We care for others but the provision for us is limited. Other groups of senior professionals such as company directors, senior lawyers and managers have their health screening sessions at BUPA Wellness or the Nuffield. I used to think these medicals were a waste of time, and medically their value is dubious in terms of revealing pathology. Having done some work on them in the past (it's enjoyable and fairly paid), I think I now realise why companies ask for them and regard them as a fairly priced maintenance cost for hard-working, stressed, senior staff who are an expensive asset to maintain. The companies who pay for these medicals are not very interested in the senior partner's hernia or ear wax or their slightly raised cholesterol. What they are keen to see is who has got stressed beyond reason, who is drinking too much, who is struggling to stay fit enough to keep up with the demanding work roles. They are a gentle way of discovering such matters and getting medical and other help in place earlier rather than later, and before the senior partner drinks away all the profits and loses all the clients. Sadly, there is no similar system in place for senior NHS doctors, although with higher rates of alcoholism and suicide than in the general population, there possibly should be.

The key point about a doctor's health is that there is the risk of a double tragedy. The sick doctor needs care and attention just like any other patient. The risk of a sick doctor is to their patients. If a doctor's illness leads to impaired performance at work, then rather than having a single tragedy we may get multiple tragedies: a sick doctor, impaired work performance, harmed patients and professional disciplinary processes activated against the doctor.

Illness and the General Medical Council

Illness may be little or no defence against disciplinary charges – the harm has happened to the patient and has to be acted upon. However, the GMC does have procedures in place to take health factors into account, and it modifies its case handling accordingly. In appraisal each year, we are asked to make a health declaration. This may seem fussy and routine but to the GMC, the old scenario of a doctor's illness not becoming apparent until the performance issue arises is no longer acceptable. The key issue for the GMC is that a doctor who has a problem is honest about it and seeks clinical and if necessary occupational health advice and treatment for it. Such a doctor shows insight, and the fact that they had had their illness treated would confirm this. The doctor who could end up in trouble at the GMC is the one who has signed off all the health declarations as 'no problems' and then when a case comes in, tries to claim illness as exculpation. Such a doctor has either put their own health at risk and not got it treated or has a dangerous lack of insight into the risk their illness poses to others. Denial and lack of insight are danger signs to those investigating medical performance issues. The health issues that most commonly catch doctors out here are drug or alcohol addiction, or severe depression.

(A brief note is needed here to remind readers that the illnesses that affect doctors most commonly are coughs, colds and backache – just as for the general British population. However, these illnesses are treatable and relatively minor, posing little risk to anyone else.)

The serious mental health conditions such as severe depression and addictions are all often hidden for many years by their sufferers. If you have one of these it is far better to get it treated than try to hide it, both for your own health and for your ability to continue in the profession.

As a doctor, I need to make sure that I am sane and healthy both for my own personal flourishing and so that I can treat patients well. When the GMC guidance starts with 'You must make care of the patient your first concern', there is a hidden presupposition that the doctor is well enough to actually do this. If you are not well enough to do this, then you need to get treatment for your own sake and for that of your patients.

The health of doctors is an issue in patient safety, and this takes concerns about our health way beyond our individual problems and concerns. We have a public persona as well as our private one. We do matter significantly to many, many others.

The stresses of medicine

The stresses of medicine are many. All doctors are to some extent wounded by their experiences as medical professionals. We all have seen sad cases, badly managed cases and difficult cases, and we have dealt with traumatic experiences. We have probably all had periods of 'relationship dysfunction' and 'poor communications' with colleagues. We will all have endured a few rows and arguments. We may have had to handle complaints against us that, no matter how baseless, still tax our patience and coping abilities. We are supposed to keep a calm, amiable and equable disposition while all around us, and maybe inside us, is a mess of seething, emotionally charged events, reactions and responses.

Now all this is of course a part of medicine, and we have to learn how to handle it, to be 'professional' and 'detached' and not to get caught up in the emotions of the situation. However, we also need to accept that medicine does make significant emotional as well as time and technical demands on its members. Yes, in the heat of medical action we have to focus on the task at hand and do the job. We cannot allow ourselves to become paralysed by emotions – we have to remain able to think and act. But every so often, we need to step back and reflect on how we handle the load of sadness, grief and stress that we encounter in our work. We are not without emotions. We are passionate and compassionate people, and our work is never merely technical. Medicine done well is never 'just business'. Our work matters to patients and our pride in doing it well is the strongest defence against bad medicine. Doing your job well is one of the best ways known of boosting your own health and self-esteem.

Therefore, we need to acknowledge the stresses of our job, and we need to put in place strategies to help us deal well with these stresses and without harm to ourselves, our families, our colleagues or our next patient. Also, as colleagues, we need to avoid harming one another. 'First do no harm' applies to colleagues as much as it does to patients.

Illness in a doctor is a personal problem for the doctor concerned, just as illness of any sort is for the patient affected. The risk of a doctor's ill health is both to the doctor as patient and to the doctor's patients. The key point about our health as doctors is to not let our ill health become a problem for others as well. As in first aid, we need to avoid the second casualty.

Tragically, many doctors have struggled on at work with severe illness, saying they are 'unable to take time off' and 'wouldn't dare to let my colleagues down' or 'show any weakness'. Many doctors still see illness as a personal failing in themselves, rather than as a problem to be dealt with. This is harsh on ourselves and, indeed, daft – most of us are actually very good at dealing with problems, once we have diagnosed them.

When we are dealing with members of the public as patients, we are professional and kind, and if they want some time away from work we usually give it to them. When we are dealing with ill colleagues, we sometimes act as if we have forgotten how to be compassionate to each other. The patient is the one with the illness and you're a doctor, not a patient. It is almost as if we cannot, or will not, cope well with the concept of 'doctor as patient', either for ourselves or in our colleagues. Sadly, if you are ill as a doctor you may find that your colleagues are not as supportive as you would like, unless you have a disastrous major pathology.

Some colleagues take a great pride in their 'presenteeism'. They are never ill and they have never had a day off sick in their lives. They sound like the old Yorkshire business owners who'd say 'I've never had a day off sick in my – (collapses)'. General John Sedgwick's classic 'They couldn't hit an elephant at this dist–' comes to mind, and we do well to retain a bit of humility in the face of the many forces of pathogenesis.

Now, the scenario I have described is readily recognisable to all of us, but the fact is that most of us do not crumple under its demands, and most of us do not succumb to stress. Most of us show resilience in our personal and professional lives. Even when we have setbacks, mostly we recover from them. We call this recovery 'experience' and even though it may be bitter, what does not kill us makes us stronger. It can be seen as a psychological version of the immune response.

All of us know that we are as vulnerable to pathology as any of our patients. Indeed, we know our vulnerabilities more – what else is medical knowledge but the catalogue of the ways in which mind and body can go bad, mad and sad? What else is life but a highly prevalent, 100% fatal, sexually transmitted illness? Like the orthopaedic surgeon's view of athletes, we come in three types: those about to get ill, those who are ill already and those recovering from illness. We know all too well how dust crumples into dust and ashes into ashes.

Handling stress

They say that stress is the tension experienced between knowing that the unreasonable person you are dealing with really needs a good thumping and knowing that you are not allowed to deliver this much-needed corrective.

Sometimes it's an inchoate rage, and you don't know who or what deserves the good kicking, but you are damn well going to find out and administer it. People help you in your enquiries, and eventually the wiser people around you point out that it is 'Roger' who (fortunately) is away for two weeks on holiday. You save your anger up for his return

117

but by then it has dissipated and you move into problem-solving mode. You smile when you see him and say 'Hello Roger. Welcome back. There was a little problem while you were away, but it's sorted now'.

Hans Selye, who defined the term 'stress' and described the autonomic responses that go with it, now admits that he used the wrong engineering metaphor. He feels he should have used the term 'strain'. Stress is the feeling we get when we are under physical and/ or mental strain.

The experience of stress is subjective: what is stressful for you may be of no concern to me. Likewise, you may wonder why I have got so stressed when the incident seems so minor to you. Stress is an outcome from an event, and our internal physiological and mental responses to that event. The events in life and work are not going to stop any time soon, so we really have to learn to deal with how we respond to events, and how we assign meaning to them. Bear in mind that the brain may assign meanings to events very quickly, and turning these reactions into considered responses may take some time. Knowing a way of hiding your immediate reactions is a useful skill in medicine. In medicine we often have to experience the stress and then deal with it later.

My colleague Dr Seth Jenkinson introduced me to a useful 'problem-solving fork'. He said that any problem can be sorted in one of four ways:

- denial
- sorting the problem
- sorting out how you respond to the problem
- moving away from the problem.

Denial is effective for a short while, at the expense of much mental effort, and sometimes absurdity when the denial becomes unsustainable. It is very commonly used, especially by government departments, as a first step in trying to deflect attention away from a problem, on the grounds that if everyone stops talking about it then it is no longer happening. Watching denial collapse into absurdity is either good fun or horrifically fascinating, depending on where you are observing from.

Sorting the problem is obviously the best answer but often you are not working at a level, or with enough position or persuasion power, to do much about it. For example, many significant event systems ask what steps the reporter has taken to prevent a recurrence. The steps needed are often not those that an individual can take, and the specific individual incident report needs considering in the context of other signals received from multiple sources. The remedial action needs to be taken at a level above the one at which the problem is experienced. Often, you just do not have the personal resources or authority to directly solve a problem.

So you then have to work on sorting out how you respond to the problem, and how you go about defining it, and working with others to sort it, and how you avoid getting frustrated with it. As a general rule, the key difference here is between a disorganised mess of misunderstood facts, high emotions and lack of organisation and a problem that emerges when you get clarity of definition and a focus on a solution, to at least part of the mess. There are whole fields that help people with this adjustment and cognitive behavioural therapy, psychology, neurolinguistic programming and many other techniques all have some successes in helping with this. Ultimately they all reach a point where you 'get your head around it'.

Moving away is sometimes a valid problem-solving option. Certain scenarios are basically insoluble and dangerous. The classic example here is the battered wife who eventually goes into a women's refuge for her own safety. There may be good reasons in certain scenarios to move away from a problem quickly. However, many people are too quick to use this option when, with persistence, a problem may eventually become soluble. Others, however, are too stubborn and they leave moving on too late, getting bogged down with a problem for too long, to their own frustration, and blocking the way for someone else to tackle it. Hitting the golden mean between these extremes is far from easy, and sometimes others may spot your predicament before you recognise or still later acknowledge it. (MSF may actually help quite a few of us here.) Very smart people know when to move on and call it 'career development'.

I could say much more about this topic but it is better at this point to direct you to the further reading at the end of this chapter and let you find your way to learning your own strategies about how to handle stress. You probably have many good ones already.

Types of stress

Medicine is intrinsically stressful. Every day, you either see stressed patients or you are stressed yourself, or both. It pays all of us to learn about coping with stress, both for ourselves and for our patients.

It is worth looking at the types of stresses we face in our work. Some stress we have to accept as part of our work. A difficult operation, an acutely ill child, seeing patients you are fond of die, breaking bad news and so on are all intrinsically stressful events that are a routine part of medicine. However, it is to be hoped that as your training has gone on, you have learned to deal with such events, such that although they are stressful, you will feel that you know how to handle them reasonably well. And you realise that sometimes the outcome will be bad, no matter how well you act. A cardiology registrar once said to me about heart failure patients, 'Yes, they do die, don't they?'. It was just what I needed to hear, and it allowed me to treat my heart failure patients more sensibly, with recognition that their prognosis was limited and that I could not stop all their deaths, and that I would not be blamed for their deaths.

The intrinsic stresses of medicine are something that we need to accept. They are part of our job and we cannot avoid them and remain as doctors.

However, much of our stress arises from other sources. Some of is internally generated. Doctors (and lawyers, and many other professionals and skilled workers) tend to be perfectionists. We want to make everything right. We want to do it in the right way, and yet we work under time and resource constraints that hinder our efforts at every turn. We can easily get frustrated that 'everything is (conspiring) against us' and 'how am I supposed to do good work when this system is so awful?'.

Perfectionists make great doctors – they are conscientious and hard-working but they can easily become stressed and highly strung, and this may tip over into depression. They work to high standards but at a personal cost. The frustrated perfectionist is a common archetype in medicine, and if you see one provoked, it's best to move out of their way until their anger has calmed. Ward sisters used to be superb at turning up with a cup of tea at just the right time to calm many a frustrated perfectionist down. GP receptionists are often good at this too. (Remember to say thank you to them after they have bailed you out.)

A lot of our stress is externally generated. They say the NHS used to be 'doctor centred' but if you call the mishmash of misaligned activities and incentives you can observe any day in a hospital or GP surgery 'doctor centred' then I wish to dispute with you. The NHS is often an inefficient monocultural monolith that sometimes runs like a tank with unoiled wheels. It sometimes steers like one too. There are a lot of frustrations in how the systems are set up to run. Why do midwives fax results to GPs rather than just issue a script themselves? Why have we not authorised and trained them to use a list of basic medicines as routine training? Why can a senior nurse not give paracetamol to a patient, while in the next bed a clueless 16 year old has administered 100 tablets to herself? Why is a nurse who can give intravenous drugs at one hospital in town not allowed to give them in the other hospital in town? Does her brain become mush as she crosses from one side to the other? Why can an item be prescribed by a GP but not by the hospital consultant? Why do doctors have to prescribe dressings and food supplements they have barely heard of rather than get the district nurses or dieticians to prescribe in their own right?

There are many, many examples of silly and frustrating systems in the NHS. Why they have not been solved years ago, I do not know. My mother (a 78-year-old retired eye surgeon) listens to me for a while and then replies 'Your father (a consultant eye surgeon from 1968 to 1990 – he died in 1999) had that problem too'. Yes, the late discharge summary and stray letter are the hardy problem weeds in the NHS garden. All NHS enquiries conclude, with the great wisdom that can only arise from profound hindsight and regret, that 'communication needs to be improved'. You would have more fun starting from the universal answer and asking, 'Now, what's the question?'.

Sometimes the world is mad, and the madness is to tolerate it. I am one of George Bernard Shaw's unreasonable men who won't. ('The reasonable man adapts himself to the world; the unreasonable one persists in trying to adapt the world to himself. Therefore, all progress depends on the unreasonable man.'[3]) Perhaps 'being reasonable' should be seen as a form of madness.

Generating health as a doctor

We have talked enough about stress in medicine. I now want to talk about how we can maintain our health and sanity as doctors. The job is as it is and like all jobs, it has its stresses, strains and madness. I doubt that as doctors we are worse frustrated perfectionists than those in other professions such as law and accountancy.

Despite the stresses of our work, most doctors are reasonably happy and reasonably healthy. Although we have some risks to our health, we are well-paid, highly intelligent professionals who have far more control over our lives than most of our fellow countrymen. Our overall mortality rates are low compared with many other professions and with lower social classes.

So how do we maintain and generate health as doctors? As I described in my paper 'Between health and illness',[4] we need to remember that health is the constantly evolving outcome from a life lived well.

How we feel on any given day is a balance between the processes of salutogenesis (health generation) and pathogenesis (disease generation). The balance between these processes is mediated by homeostasis.

In this section I want to look at what helps generate health for us. Wealth is the first thing to mention. Wealth and health derive from similar roots. As the study of health inequalities shows, the richer you are, the healthier you are and the longer you live. There's a strong correlation between education and wealth-generating ability. So being well educated gets you good jobs that generate wealth, and tend to leave you healthier. As a doctor, you start from here.

Second, respect and esteem generate health. We are social animals and we cannot live fully free of the good or bad opinions of others. As doctors, we get a lot of recognition from our colleagues and our patients. Getting additional qualifications such as a Master's degree or your college fellowship is a good esteem boost.

Third, physical fitness is helpful – fitter people think more clearly and withstand stress better. Their cardiovascular system is stronger.

Fourth, resilience is the antidote to stress. We look a lot at stress but most of us do not buckle under it. Human beings are resilient and able to withstand many stresses successfully.

Fifth, relationships are helpful. You can never be too good at relating to your family, your children and your colleagues – and, one would hope, a few friends from other activities. Relationships with friends generate health. Appropriate use of mood alteration strategies is useful. These can all be underdone or overdone but if they are done to the right amount, they can be helpful.

- Advisable – sex, exercise, religious activities, group activities, alcohol, coffee, chocolate, salt, food, antidepressants, thrill seeking (e.g. rock climbing), relaxation, writing, hobbies.

- Inadvisable – illegal drugs, drunkenness, crime, fights, smoking, too much of the advisable activities, overtraining, driving too fast, installing wife number 2 and hoping wife number 1 won't mind, having an affair with the practice nurse.

Sixth, a sense of coherence – a sense that things make sense, that we have a place and a role in the world and that we can make some difference by our actions. This leads on to a sense of personal effectiveness. If the revalidation system works as we hope it will, it will help us build our sense of personal effectiveness.

Seventh, a sense of humour is useful. In medicine we see a lot of the absurd; we see many versions of Sisyphus pushing heavy burdens uphill only for those same burdens to flatten Sisyphus as they roll back downhill. We know that all efforts are ultimately futile. Somewhere along the way, we must find a source of meaning and purpose for our lives, either a religious system or, as Sartre described for the atheists, we must make our own version.

Eighth, being involved is important. The elements already mentioned combine to leave you in a healthy place from which it becomes natural to be involved in whatever activity you choose. The activity is likely to have purpose, and to lead to many other relationships that make life interesting and allow you to learn much more from others. Sartre said that 'hell is other people'. We need to remember that so too is heaven. My basic belief is that the more interesting people I can meet, the more fun I will have and the more learning I will enjoy.

So we can see the elements we need to have in place that should help us stay sane, healthy and resilient. Finally, remember the Oslerian wisdom of 'Normal? Normal? What do you mean normal? The only person who's fully normal is the one we haven't examined properly'. Marry that up with Jung's insight: 'Show me a sane man and I will cure him for you'. We are none of us entirely normal, and we all have our oddities.

As someone has suggested, 'an eccentric has learned to be happy with their neuroses, while the neurotic is still unhappy with their eccentricities'.

To your good health.

References

1 Davies P, Moran L, Gandhi H. In: *The New GP's Handbook*. London: Radcliffe Publishing; 2012.
2 Shem S. The fat man. In: *The House of God*. London: Bodley Head; 1978.
3 Shaw B. *Maxims for Revolutionists*. Project Gutenburg. 1903.
4 Davies P. Between health and illness. *Perspect Biol Med*. 2007; **50**(3): 444–52.

Further reading

- Bennet G. *The Wound and the Doctor: healing, technology and power in modern medicine*. London: Secker & Warburg; 1987.
- Ghodse H, Mann S, Johnson P, editors. *Doctors and their Health*. Sutton, Surrey: Reed Business Information; 2000.
- Rowe L, Kidd M. *First Do No Harm: being a resilient doctor in the 21st century*. Maidenhead: McGraw-Hill Medical; 2009.
- Siebert A. *The Resiliency Advantage: master change, thrive under pressure, and bounce back from setbacks*. San Francisco, CA: Berrett-Koehler; 2005.

Sources of help for sick doctors

If you are currently a sick doctor the following sources of help may be useful to you either in terms of treating your illness or helping you with the effects the illness has on your work.

- Your GP – the first point of entry to the NHS

- Your medical director – they will want to know about the problem and if they are involved early they will respect your insight and help you get right again, which is good for you and allows them to protect patient safety. They may be MDs but they are doctors first and foremost. And if you conceal a problem from them, they will be unimpressed

- Occupational health service – often very good at mediating between your needs and the requirements of your work, and getting a good solution into place

- Your BMA or LMC – often good at managing the employment side of things

- The Sick Doctor's Trust – www.sick-doctors-trust.co.uk (accessed 17 December 2012)

- HOPE – www.hope4medics.co.uk/support.php (accessed 17 December 2012)

- Support for Doctors – www.support4doctors.org (accessed 17 December 2012)

- BMA Doctor Support Service – http://bma.org.uk/practical-support-at-work/doctors-well-being/doctor-support-service (accessed 17 December 2012)

- Practitioner Health Programme (London) – http://php.nhs.uk (accessed 17 December 2012)

If you are a sick doctor get help early, and before the illness damages you, your family or your patients. *DO IT NOW.*

Index

CPD with Radcliffe

You can now use a selection of our books to achieve CPD (Continuing Professional Development) points through directed reading.

We provide a free online form and downloadable certificate for your appraisal portfolio. Look for the CPD logo and register with us at: **www.radcliffehealth.com/cpd**

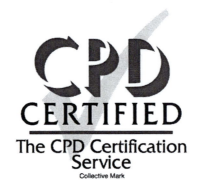

CPD
CERTIFIED
The CPD Certification
Service
Collective Mark